Vaccinate

Visit worldsofconnections.com/covid-vaccine-posters to download the posters in this book at no cost. The Vaccinate Project is supported by the Worlds of Connections SEPA (Science Education Partnership Award) [R25GM129836] and the Worlds of Connections: Vaccine Hesitancy SEPA Administrative Supplement [3R25GM129836-04S1] at the University of Nebraska–Lincoln, funded by the National Institute of General Medical Sciences of the National Institutes of Health. The content herein and on worldsofconnections.com is solely the responsibility of the creators and does not necessarily represent the official views of the National Institutes of Health or the University of Nebraska.

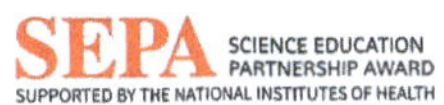

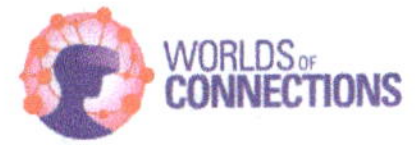

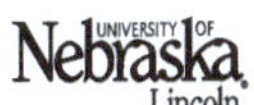

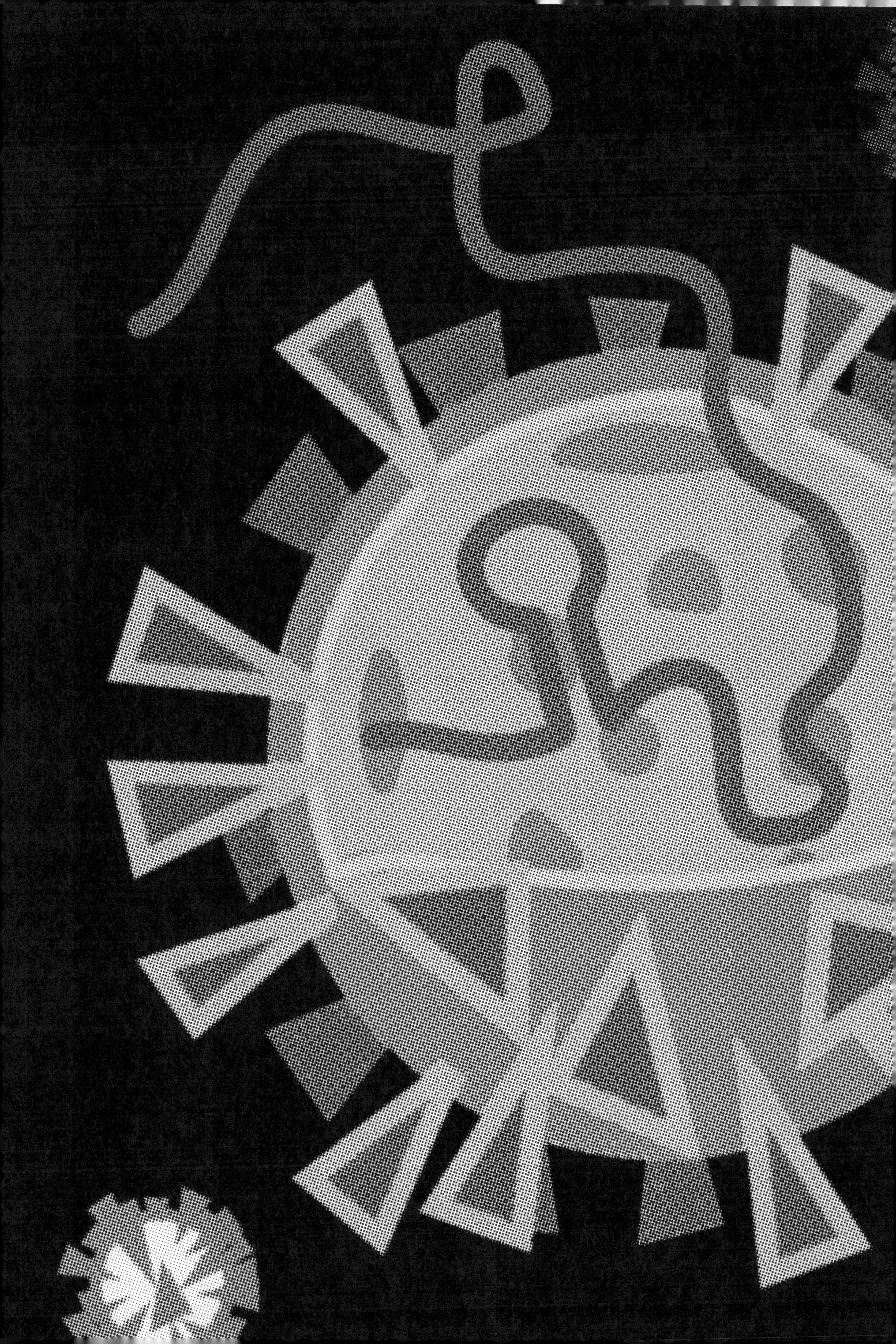

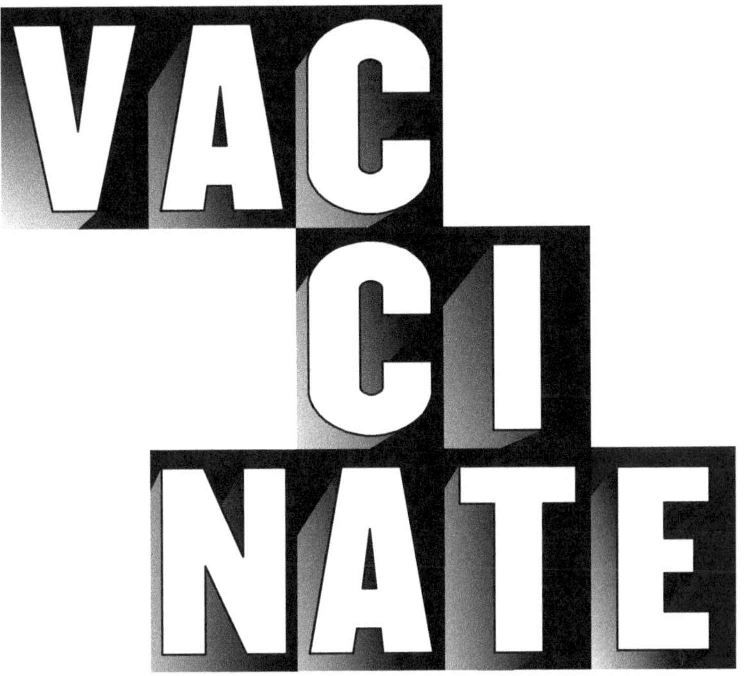

Posters from the COVID-19 Pandemic

Curated by Aaron Sutherlen, Judy Diamond, Meghan Leadabrand, and Julia McQuillan

Foreword by St Patrick Reid

Introduction by Julia McQuillan, Judy Diamond, and Meghan Leadabrand

Book design by Aaron Sutherlen

ZEA BOOKS
LINCOLN, NEBRASKA
2022

Library of Congress Control Number: 2022942070

ISBN 978-1-60962-266-4 paperback
ISBN 978-1-60962-267-1 ebook
DOI:10.32873/unl.dc.zea.1334

Zea Books are published by the University of Nebraska–Lincoln Libraries.

Electronic (pdf) edition available online at
https://digitalcommons.unl.edu/zeabook/

Art is science

Science is art

Never to be untangled

Or appreciated with any level of hesitancy

That is the only way faith and hope can persist

In both a spiritual and quantum way

As Basquiat had the cat the whole time

Art is science

Science is art

Never to be untangled

St Patrick Reid PhD
Pathology and Microbiology
University of Nebraska Medical Center

Introduction

Why Ask Artists to Help Reduce Vaccine Hesitancy?

By Julia McQuillan, Judy Diamond, and Meghan Leadabrand

In 2022 we are living through a global pandemic, and vaccines are one of the most effective strategies for slowing the spread of infectious disease, minimizing symptoms, and lowering healthcare demands. In short, vaccines save lives and can reduce the risk of contagion from social interaction.

Science and medicine have coalesced to improve the health of many people. For example, anesthesia controls pain, insulin adjusts human hormones to control diabetes, robotic-assisted surgeries shorten healing time, and better understanding of human genetics has led to recognition of specific disease-causing cells and thus better cancer therapies. The creation of vaccines is arguably the most remarkable of all scientific and medical discoveries. By working with the human immune system, vaccines reduce the spread and lower the damage of diseases caused by viruses. Each year vaccines prevent four to five million deaths from infectious diseases such as measles, polio, rabies, tetanus, cholera, typhoid, yellow fever, tuberculosis, diphtheria, hepatitis, influenza, human papillomavirus, and meningitis.

The COVID-19 pandemic spread like wildfire, catching much of the world unprepared to protect people from sickness and death. In the midst of chaos, scientists collaborated to build on decades of discoveries that led to rapid vaccine creation against severe acute respiratory syndrome coronavirus 2 (SARS-CoV-2). We may not want to remember much from a pandemic that resulted in over six million deaths, but never before in the history of medicine had an effective prevention against deadly disease been so quickly refined, manufactured, and made broadly available.

In the United States in late 2021, after the vaccines had been broadly available for almost a year, one in five adults still chose not to get vaccinated against COVID-19. Most scientists and medical experts are perplexed that people are hesitant about or simply reject life-saving vaccines. Millions remain unprotected against infection by the COVID-19 virus, and for many reasons. Some people were infected and/or died before the vaccine was available, others are too immunocompromised to get the vaccine, and, for a very few, the vaccine is insufficient. Others do not benefit from vaccination because of political messaging, gaps in social infrastructure, religious concerns, misinformation, and lack of trust—in part based upon historical evidence—that government-supported science and medicine will act in their best interests. Some, including many young people, assume that COVID-19 is primarily a disease of the elderly. Others fear that the vaccine is more dangerous than the disease it protects against. Regardless of the concerns, the high rates of vaccine rejection in the United States put it at odds with most of the world's other developed countries, where vaccination rates are much higher.

We had the opportunity to invite artists to join this project as part of a supplement grant to our National Institutes of Health–funded initiative, Worlds of Connections. After our team sought submissions during fall 2021, a committee of six advisors, with backgrounds in epidemiology, public health, veterinary medicine, sociology, graphic art, and comic art, selected 34 out of 66 pieces. We commissioned 10 additional works from comic artist Bob Hall, who was the lead artist of *C'RONA Pandemic Comics* (University of Nebraska Press 2021), and two from Ho-Chunk multidisciplinary artist Henry Payer. The submissions are the handiwork of artists from across the United States, plus one from Mexico. They come from artists young and old, from many walks of life and diverse professions.

Art can disrupt what is embedded in our minds and open us up to new perspectives and insights. We hope to offer access to images, insights, and knowledge that help people have the freedom to consider their role in the pandemic and the role of vaccines. We hope that experiencing the creativity, humor, and sentiments of artists will encourage those who have avoided the COVID-19 vaccine to reconsider and take advantage of a way to prepare their immune system should they be exposed to the virus. We are thrilled to provide the posters for those who want to enjoy, reflect, and share them with others who are inspired by the power of vaccines and who want to help stop the spread of deadly viruses.

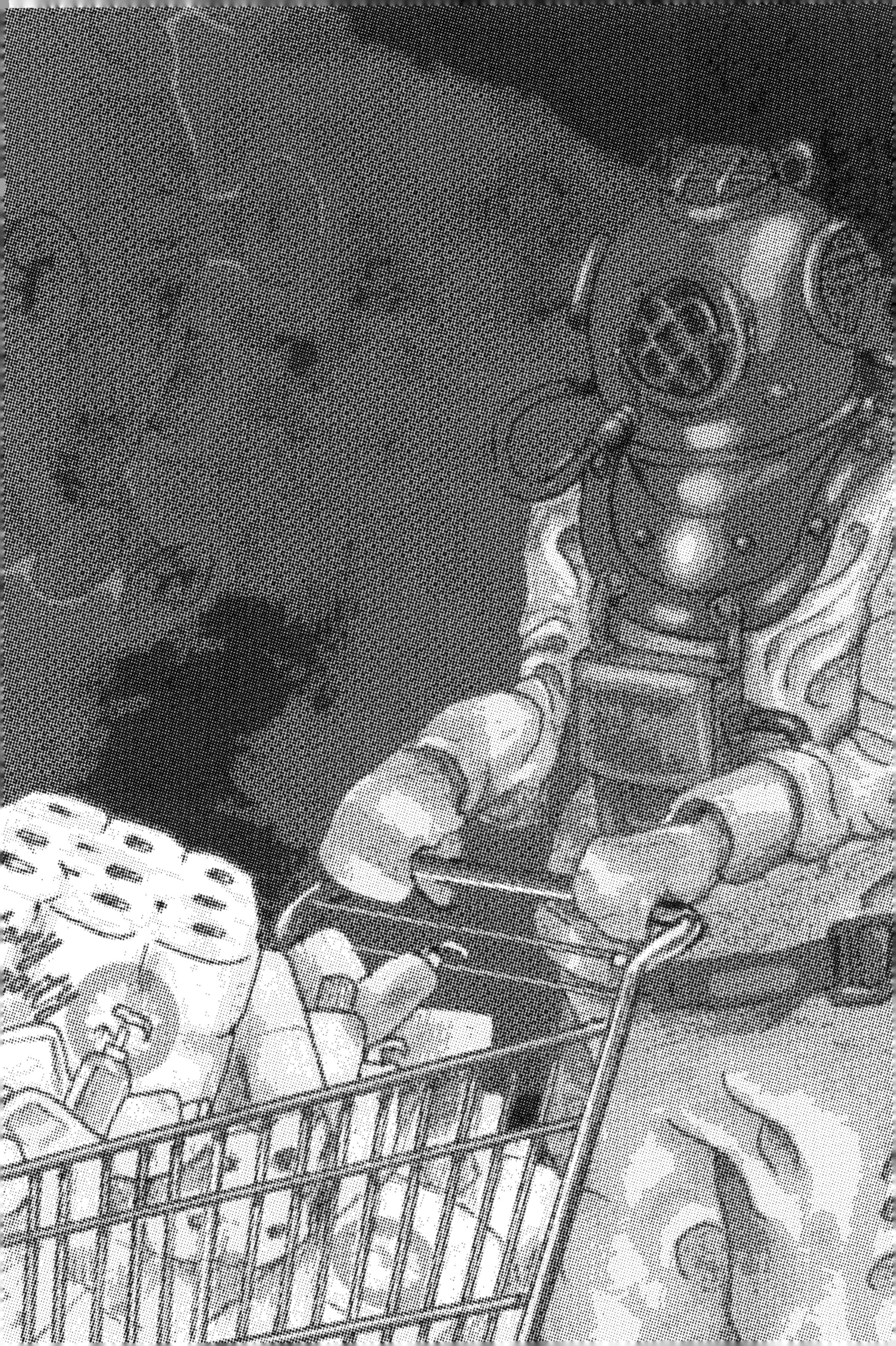

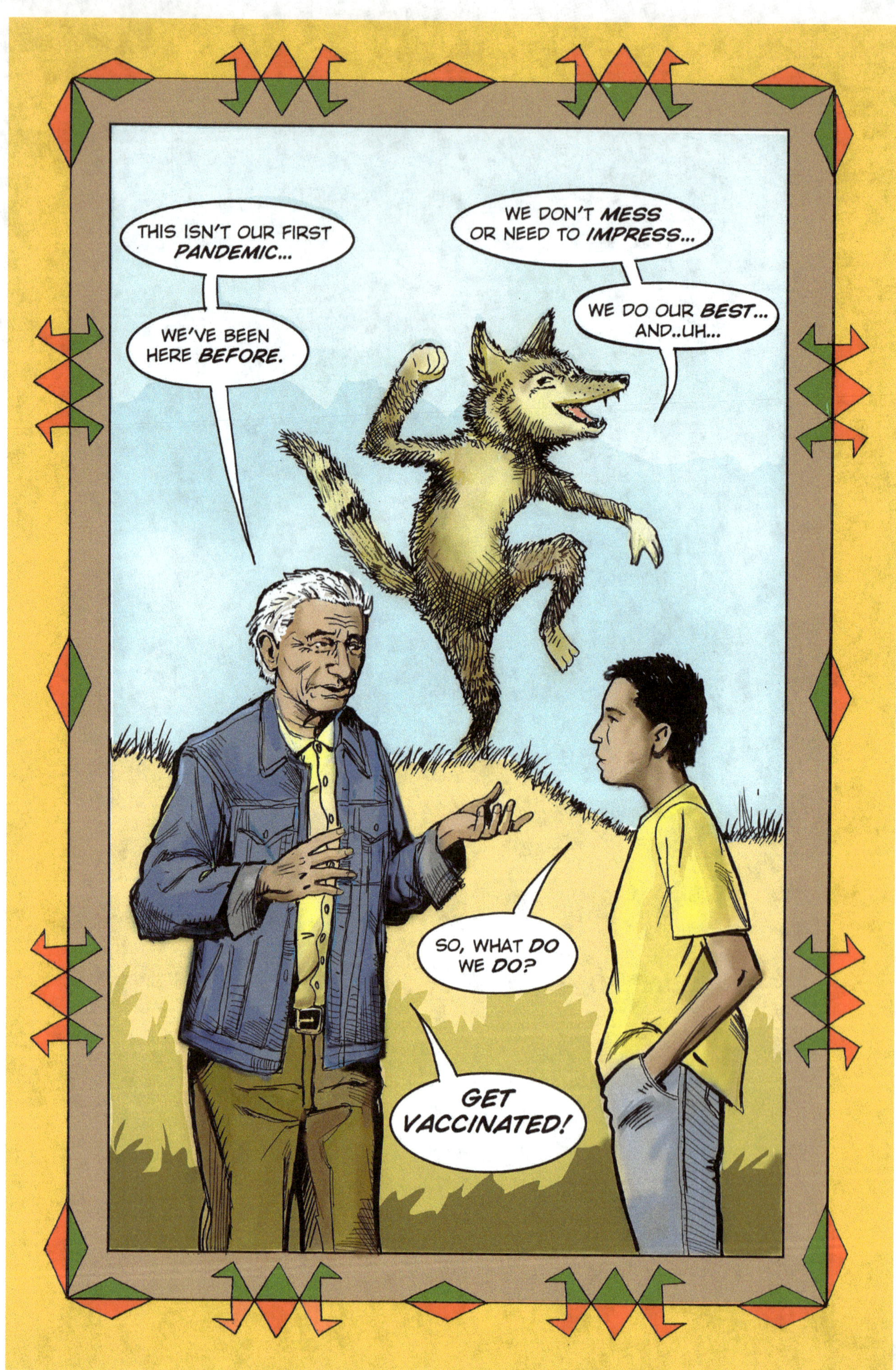

Art by Henry Payer and Bob Hall.

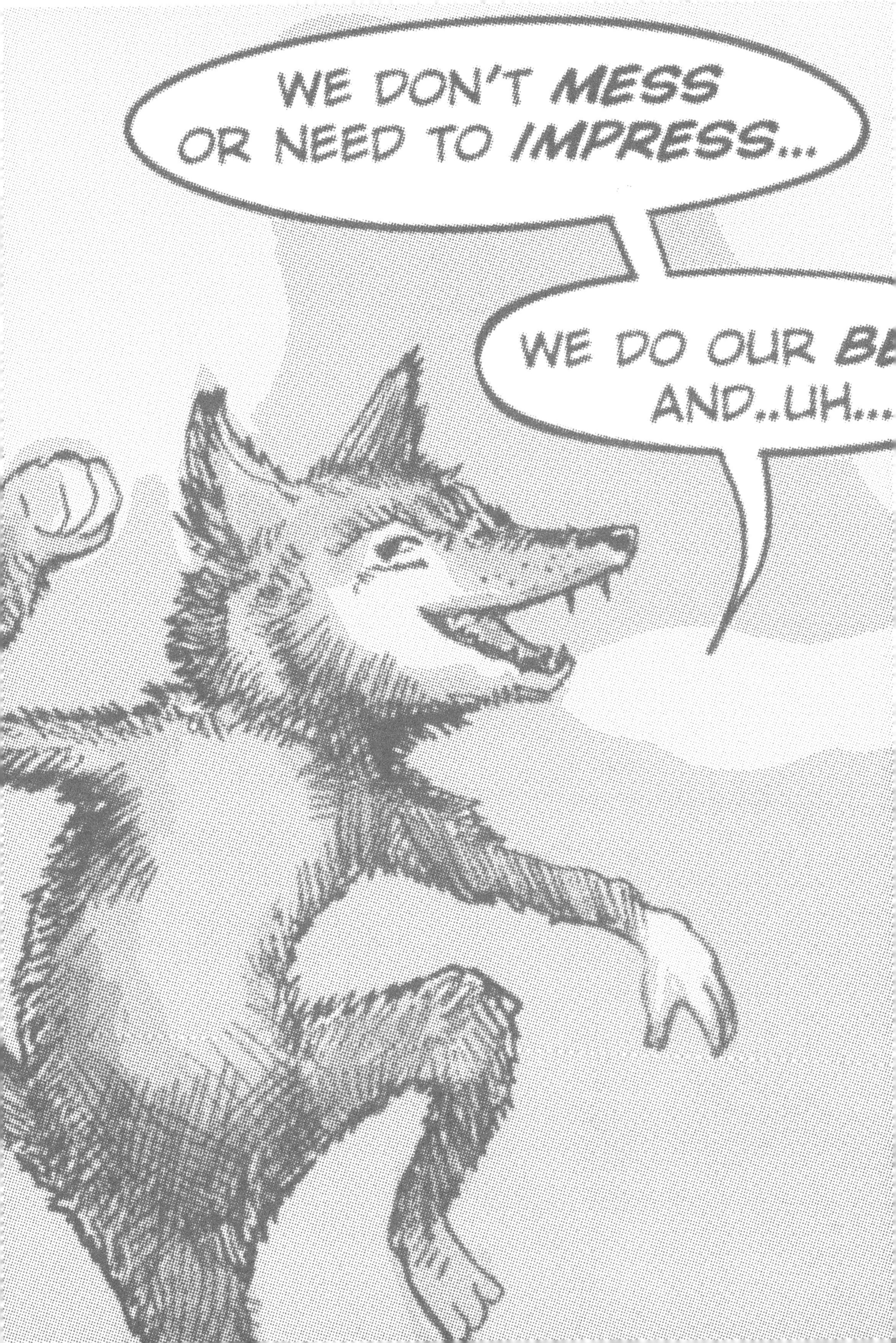
WE DON'T *MESS* OR NEED TO *IMPRESS*...
WE DO OUR *B*
AND..UH...

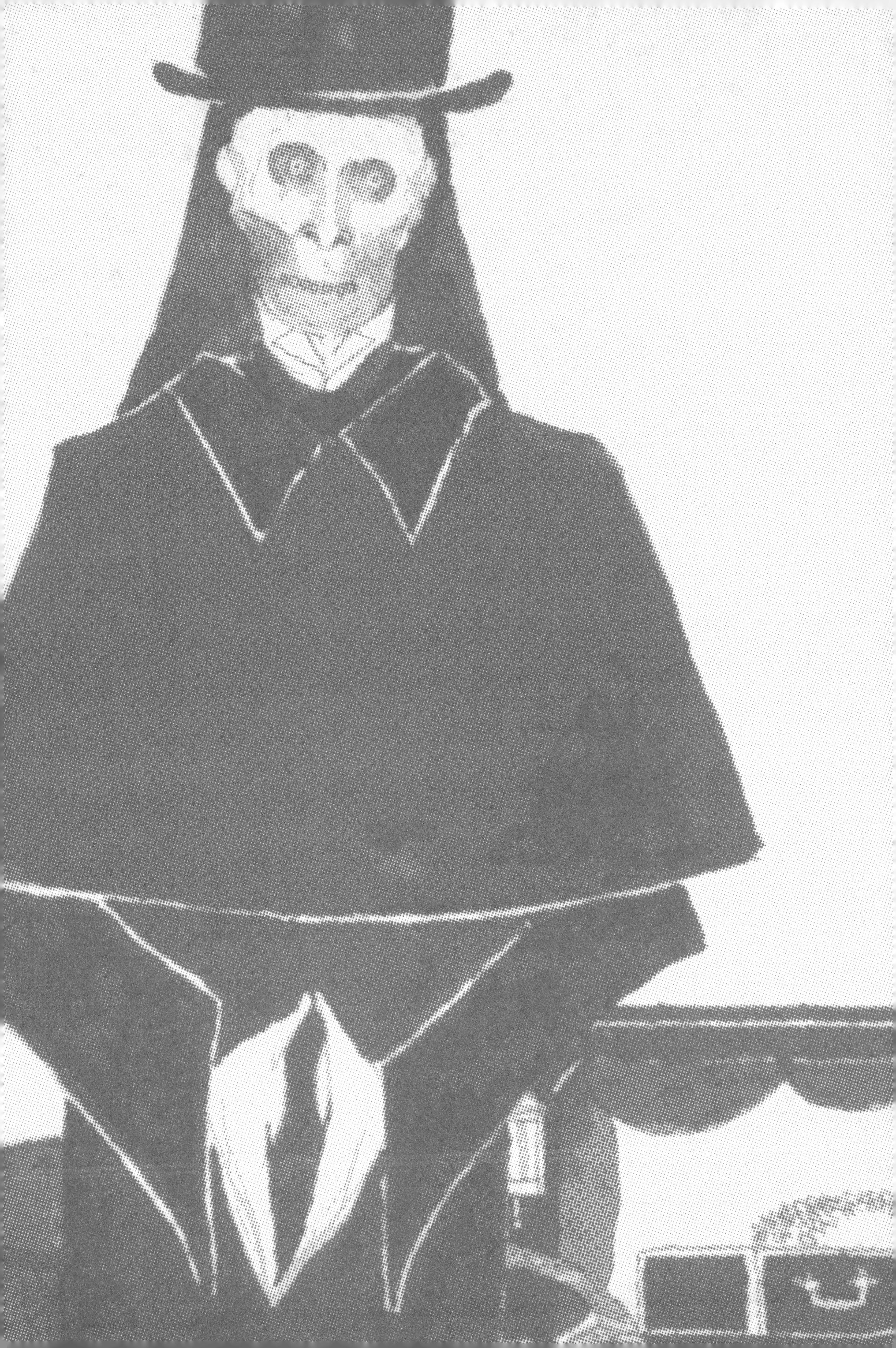

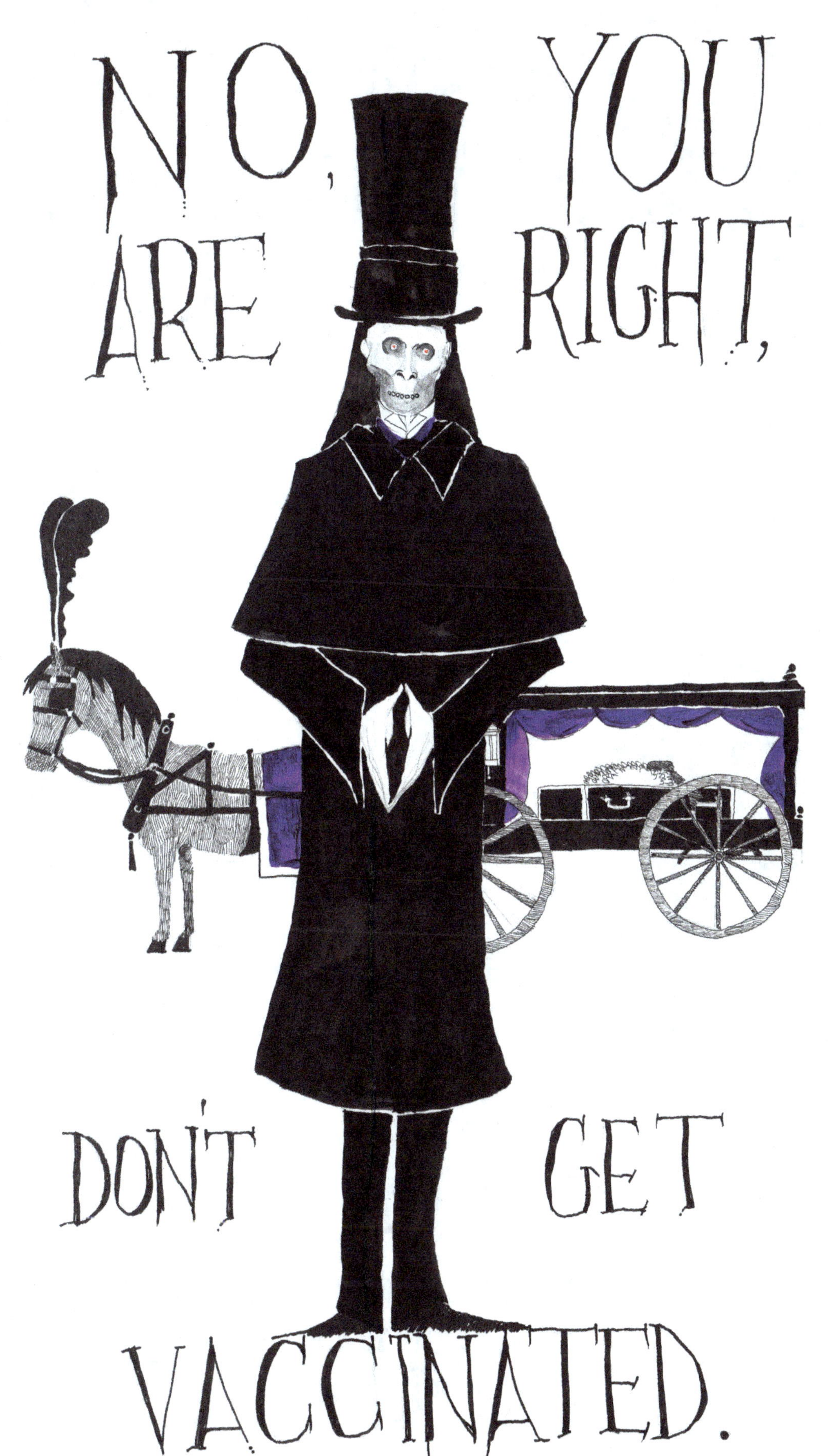

Art by Stephen Lahey.

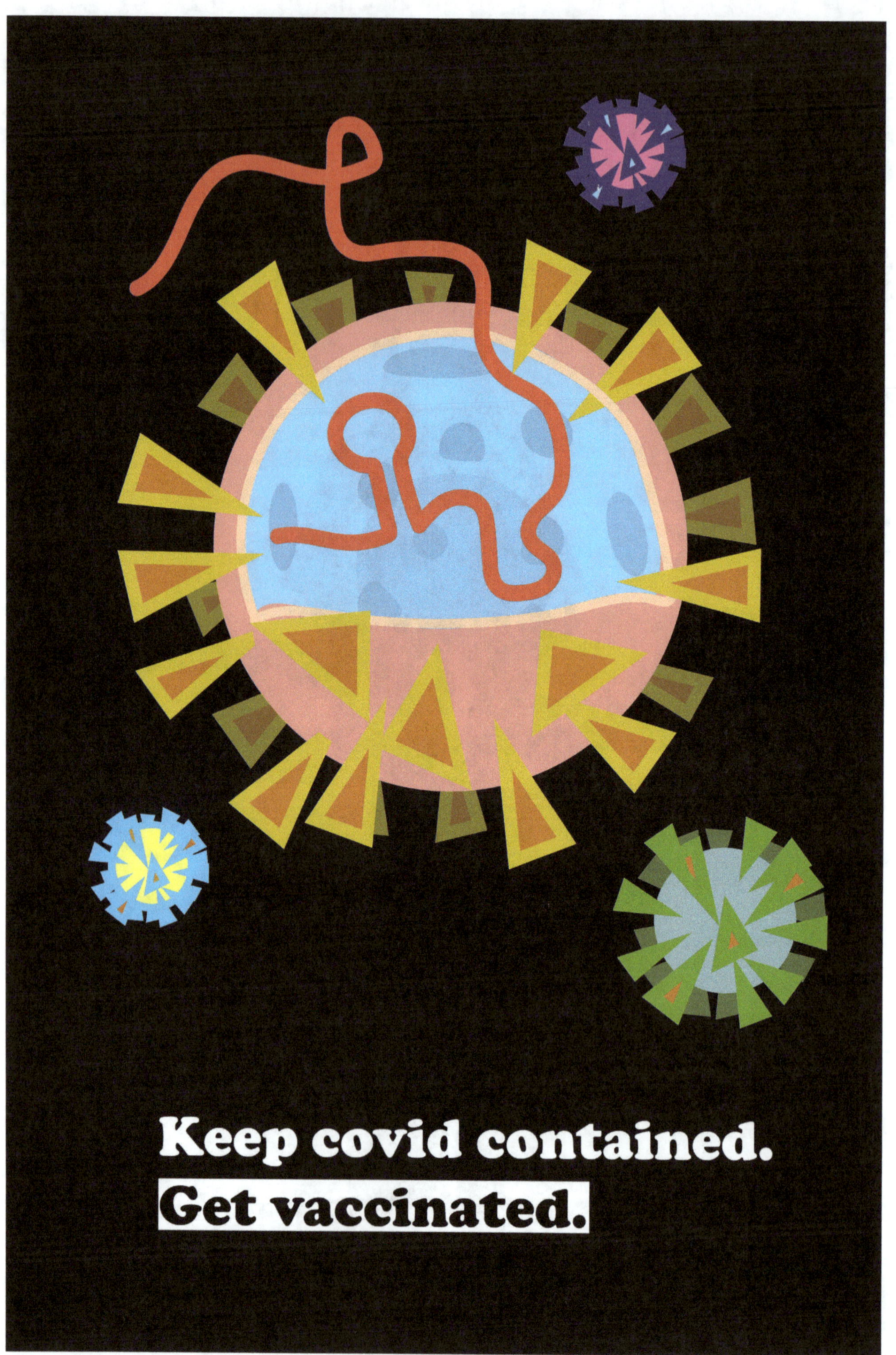

Art by Nicholas Deason.

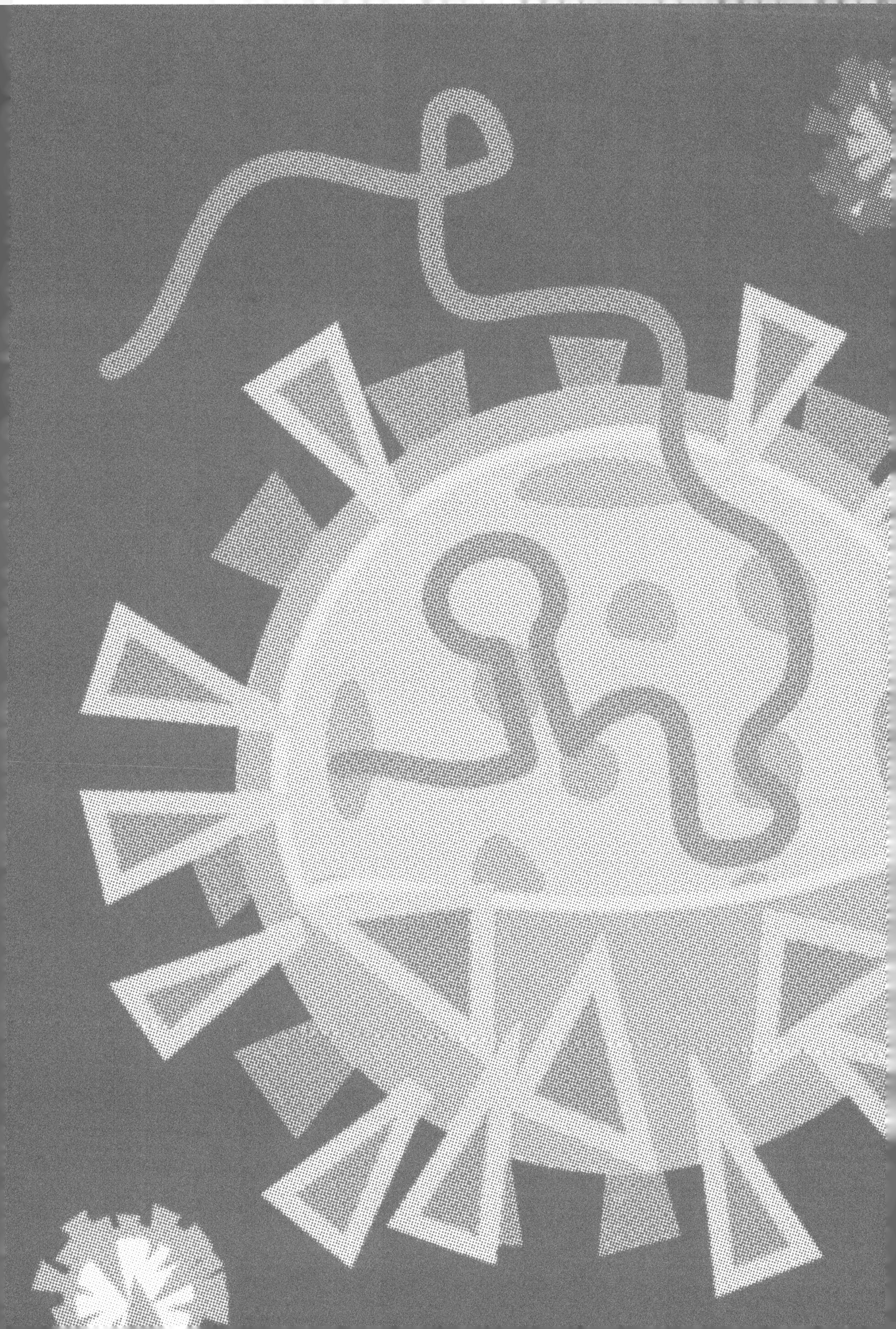

at them before...

Polio

Smallpo

Whoo

We'll beat the

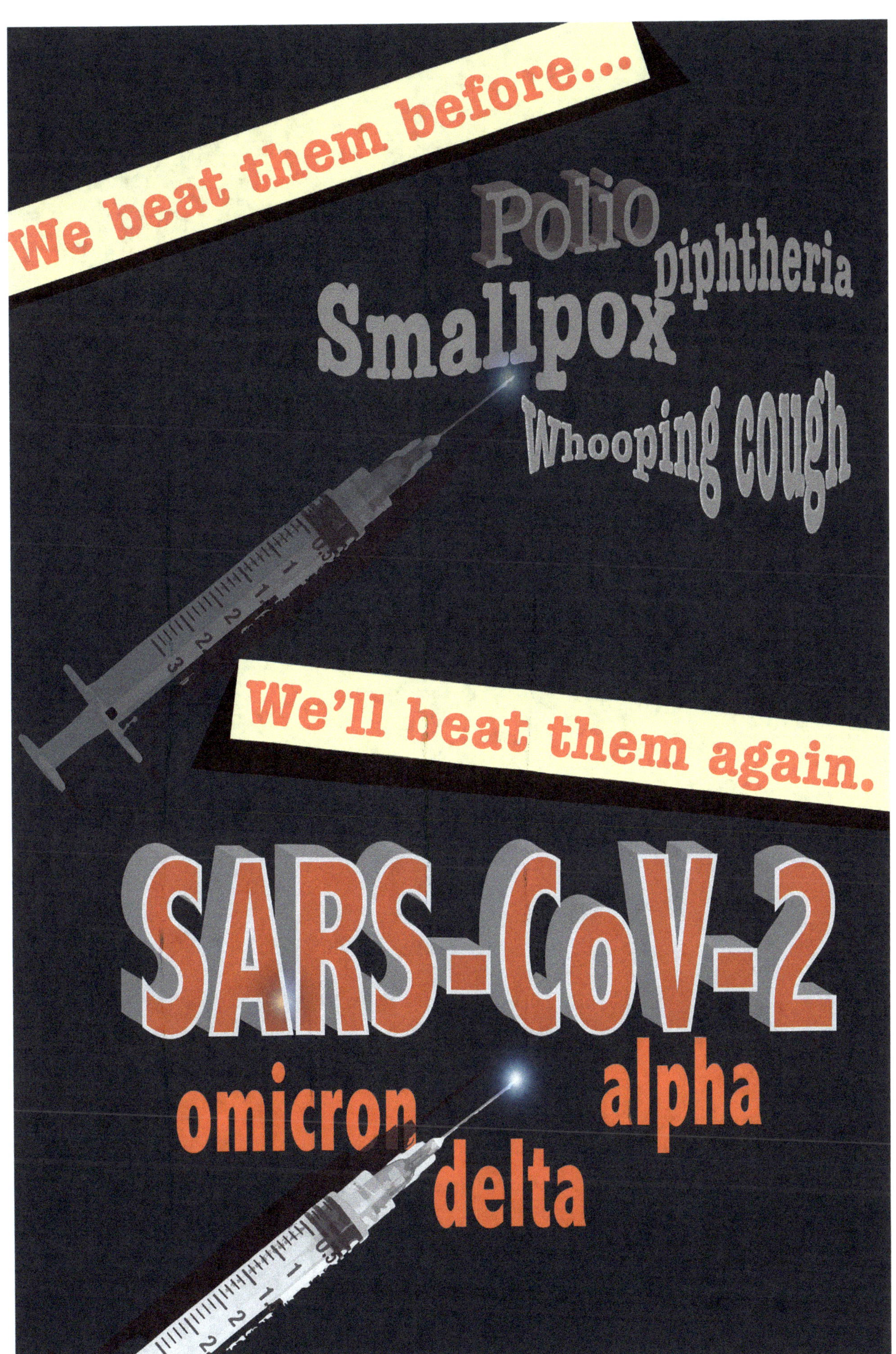

Art by Nicholas Deason.

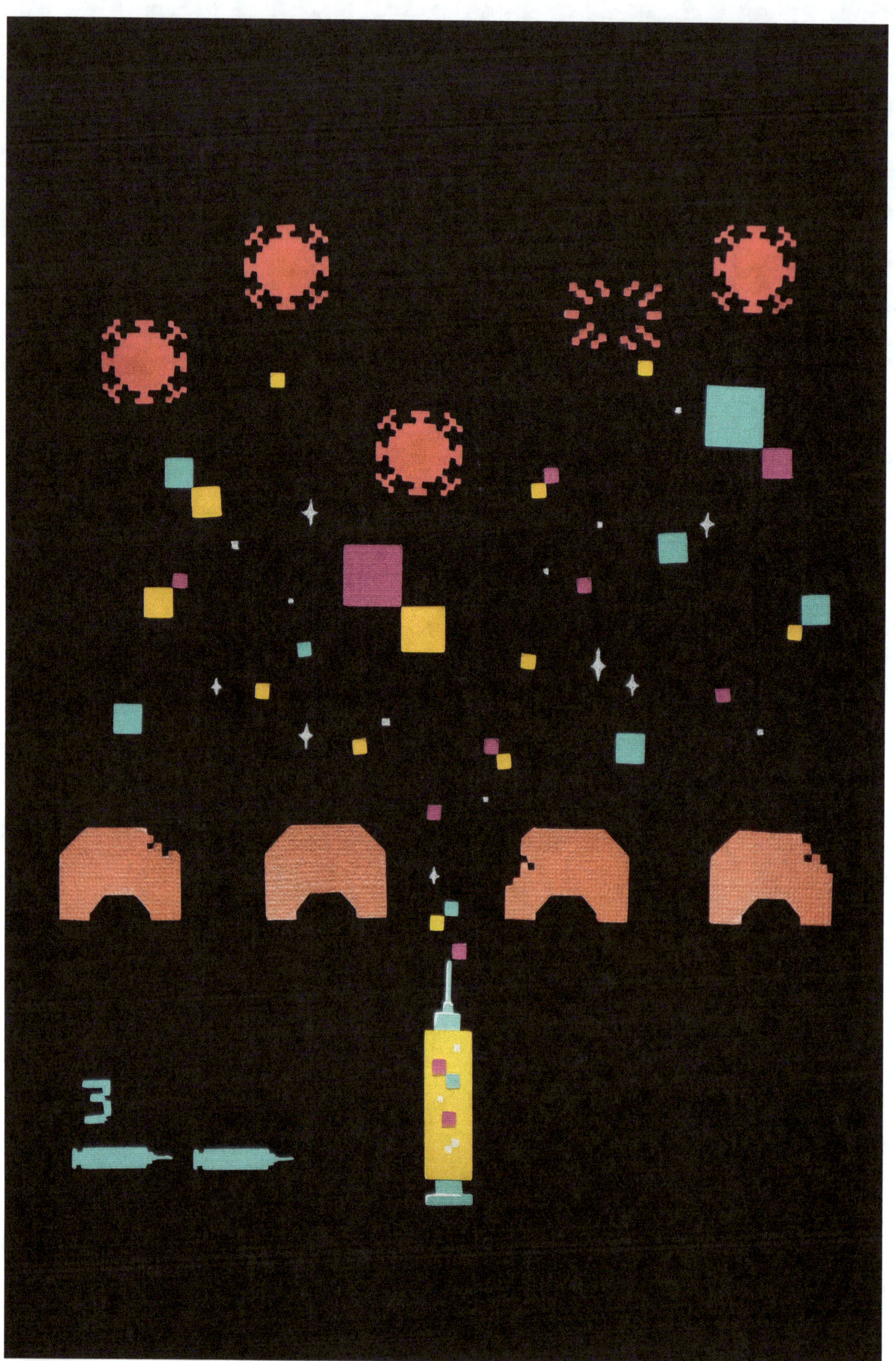

Art by Katie Nieland.

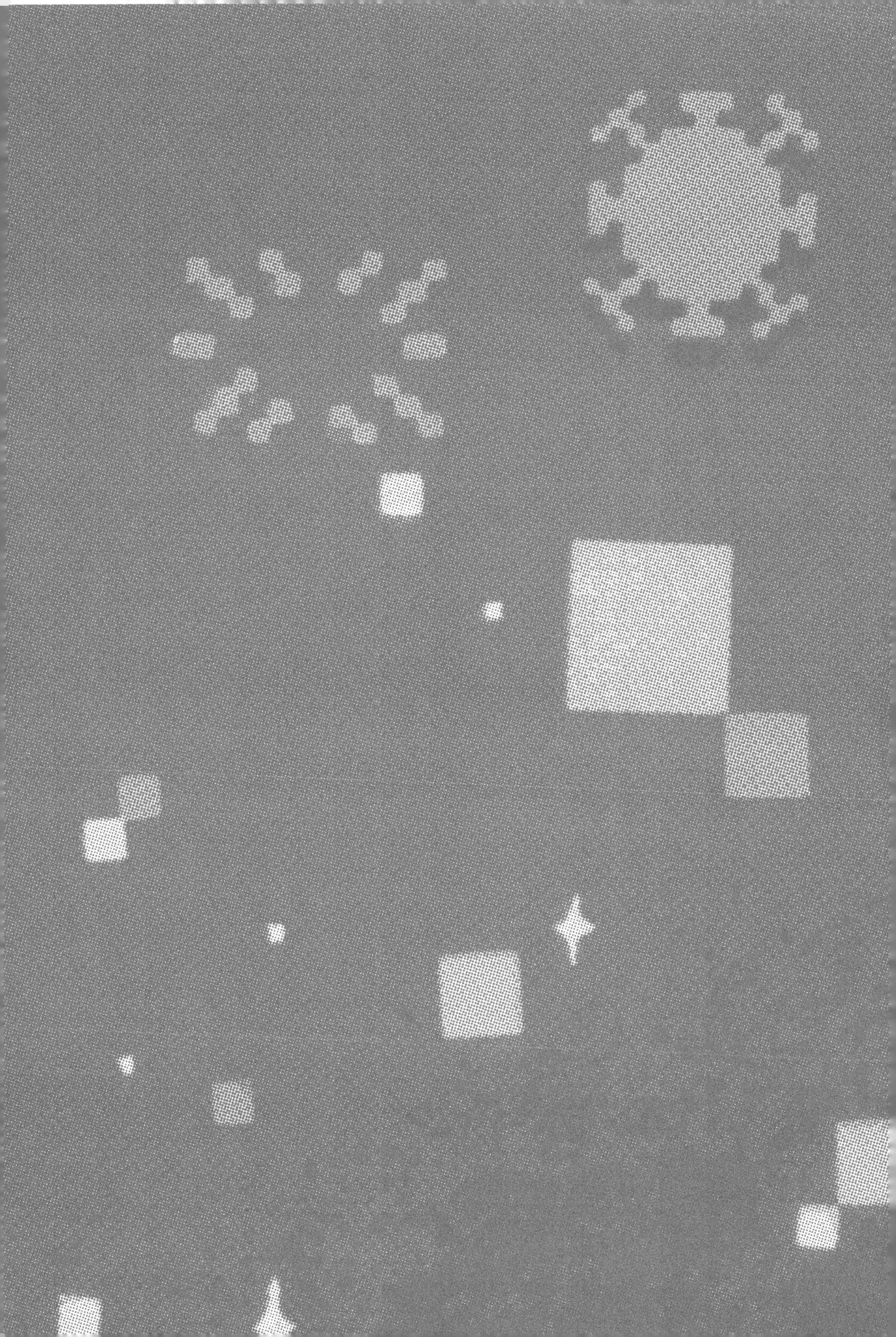

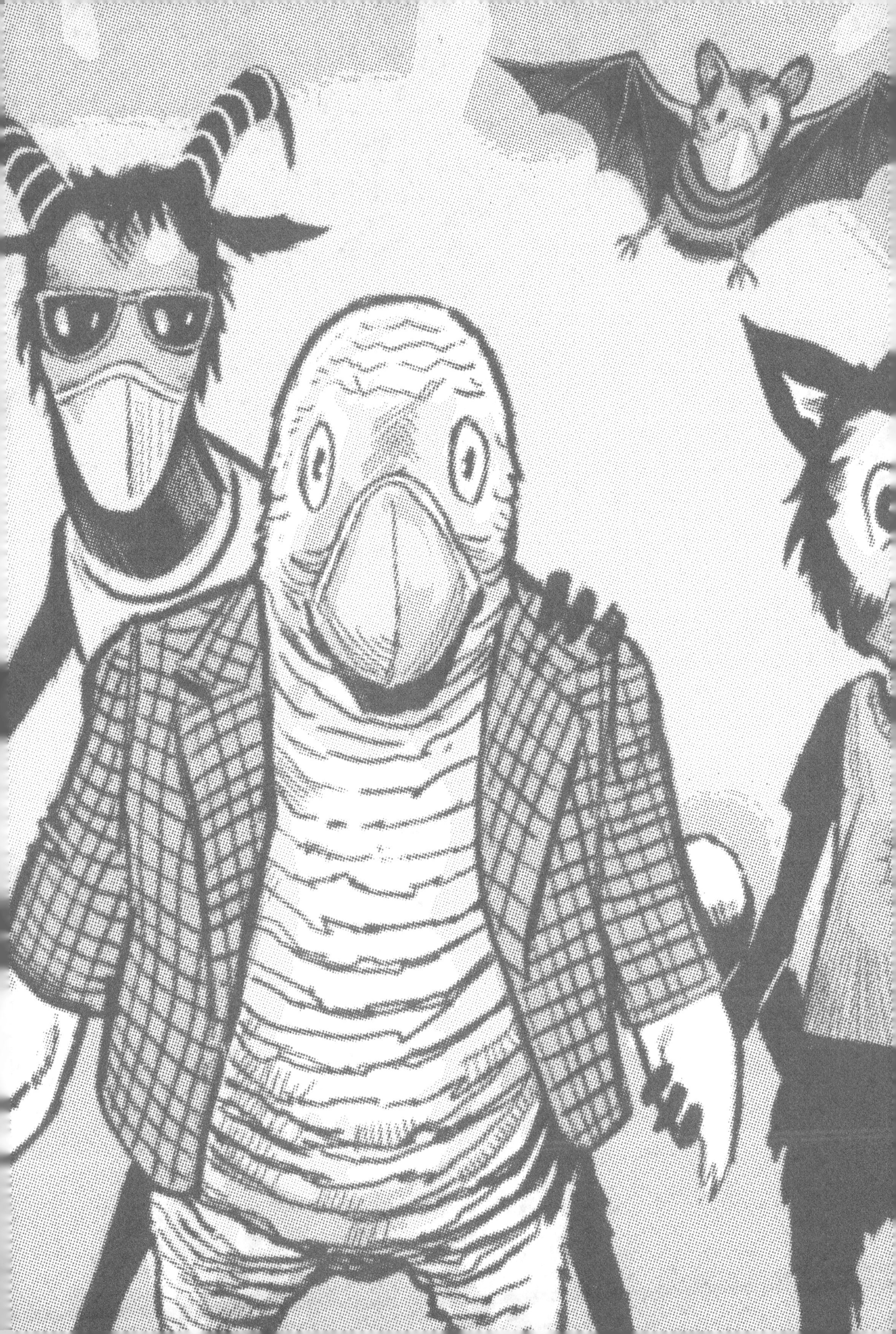

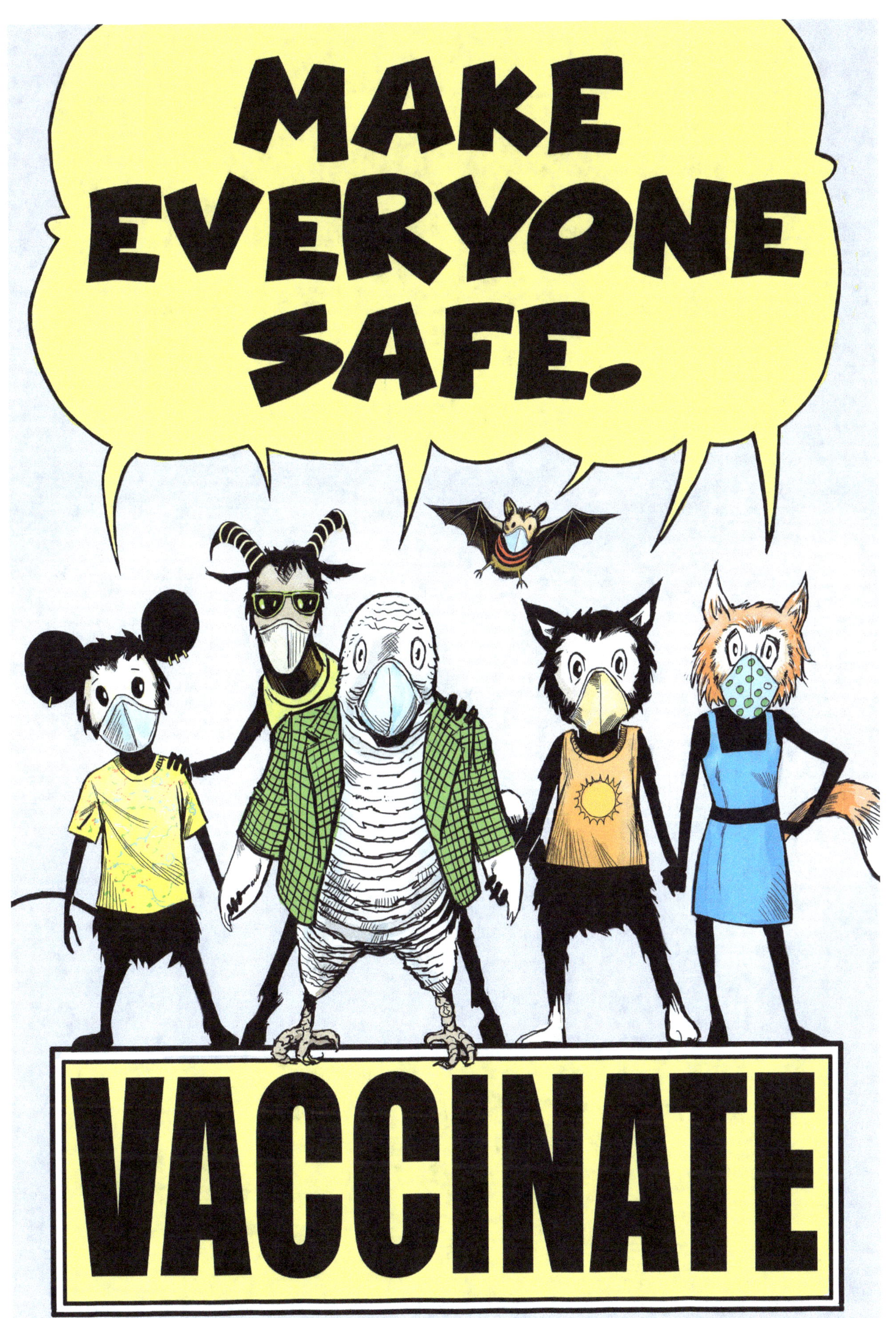

Art by Bob Hall.

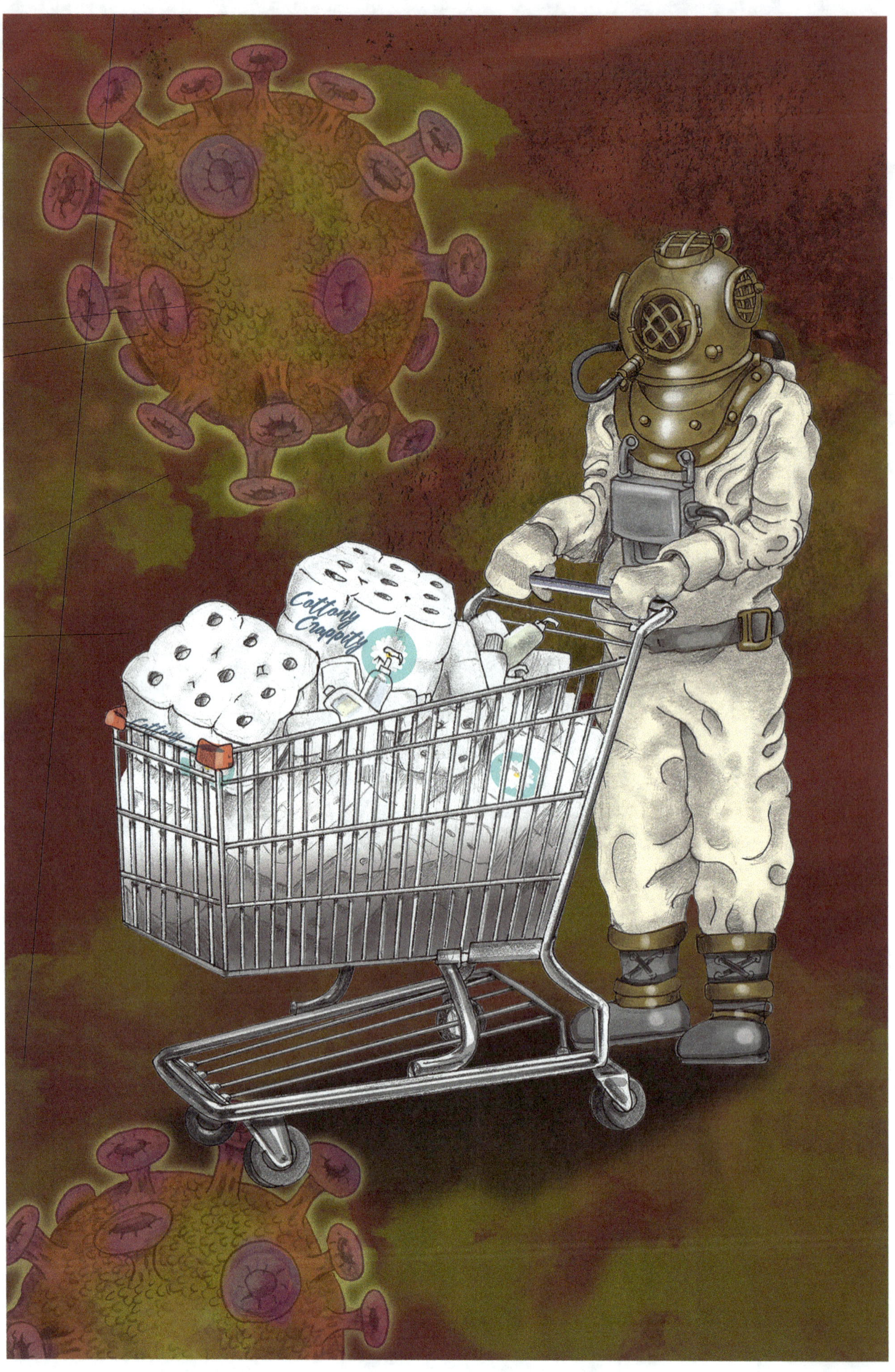

Art by Pawl Tisdale.

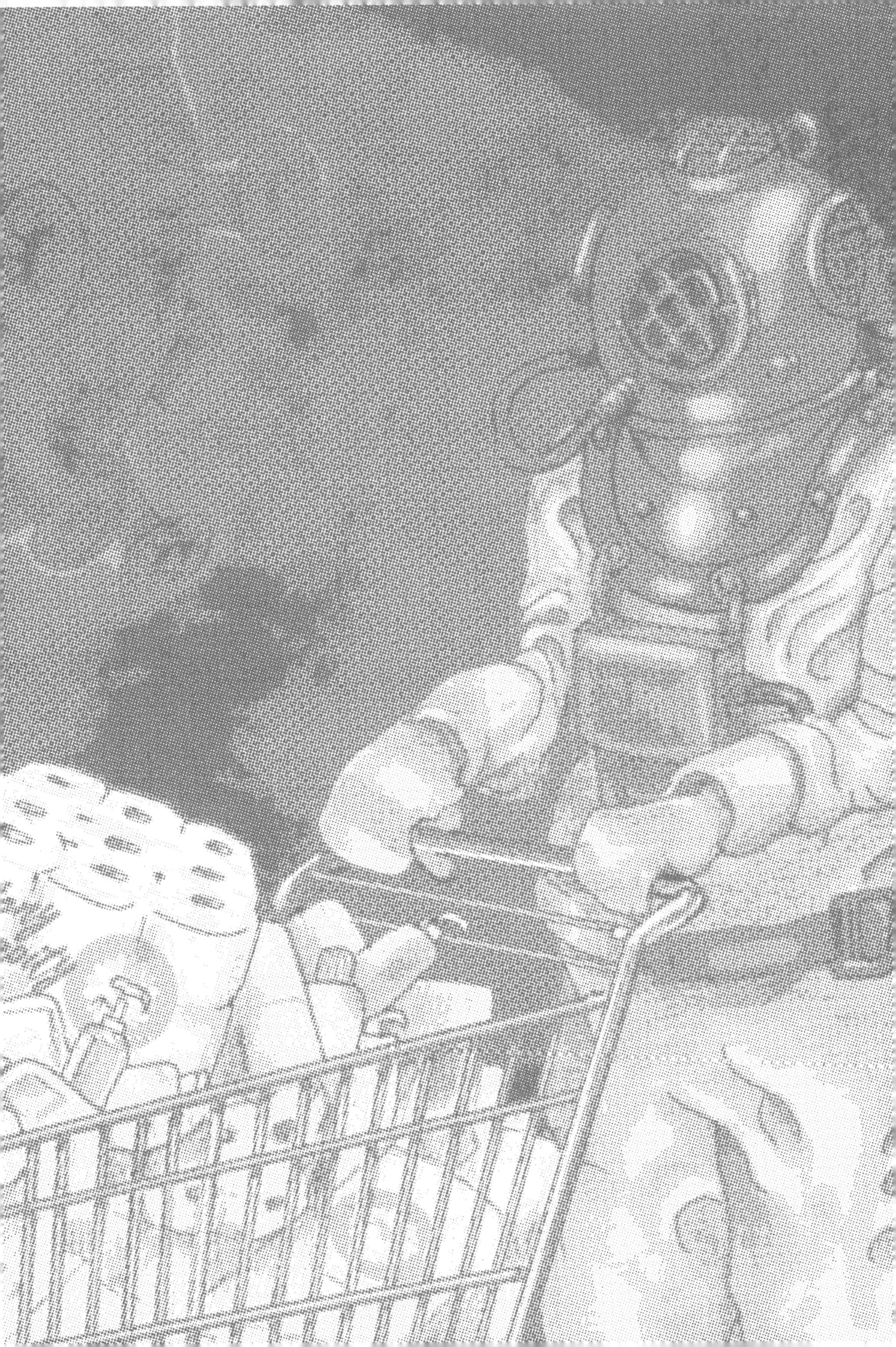

LIBRARY OF DISEASE DISGUISES

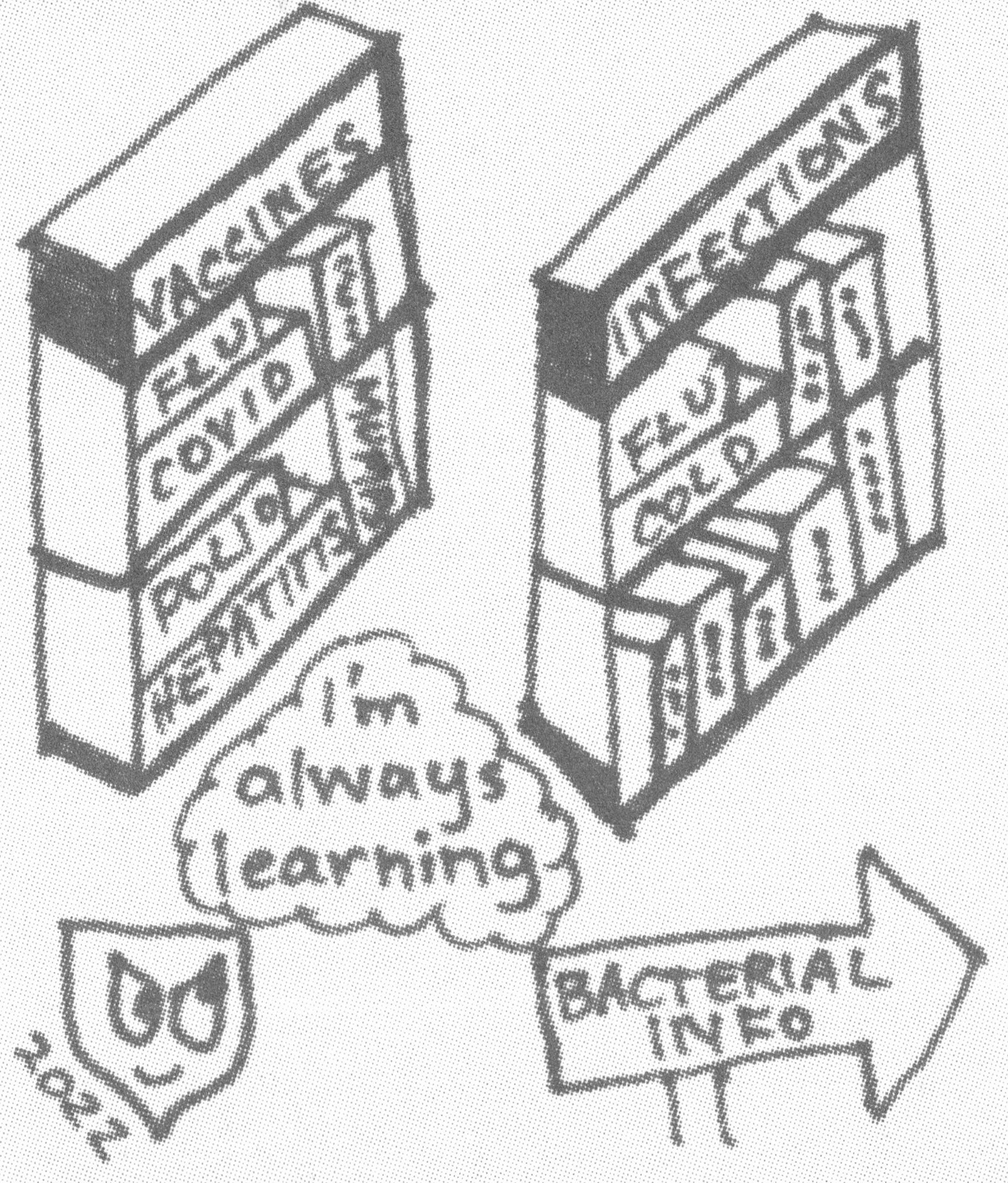

A BOOK I READ ABOUT THE 1918 FLU PANDEMIC MADE ME WANT TO GET ALL THE VACCINES I CAN.

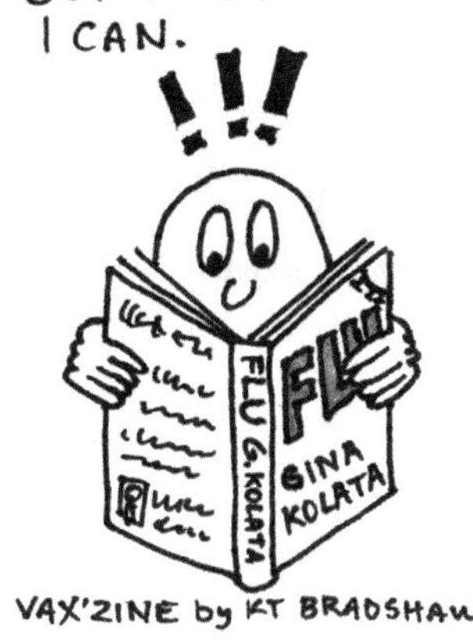

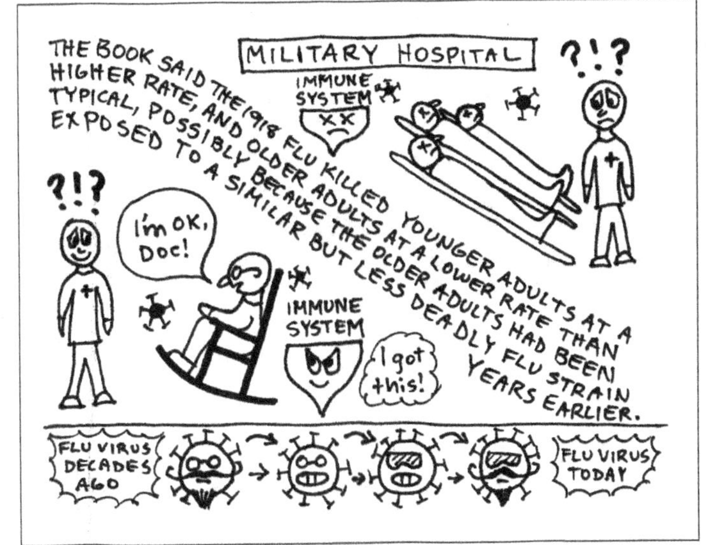

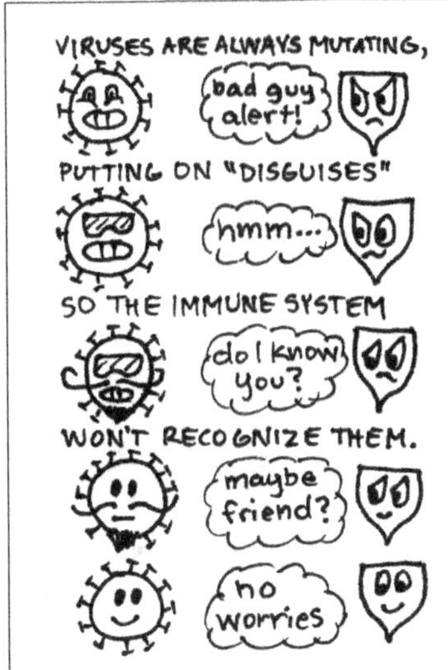

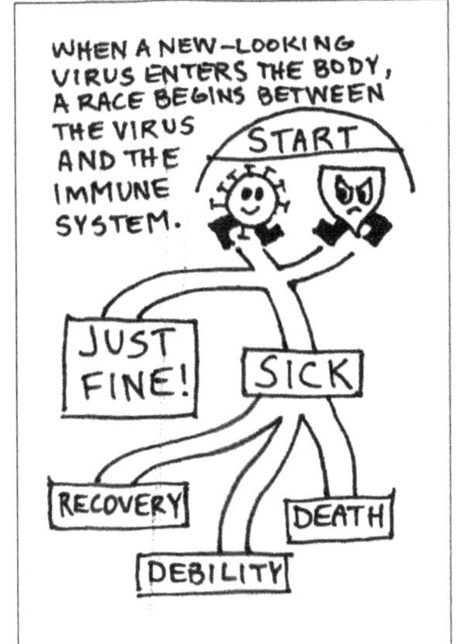

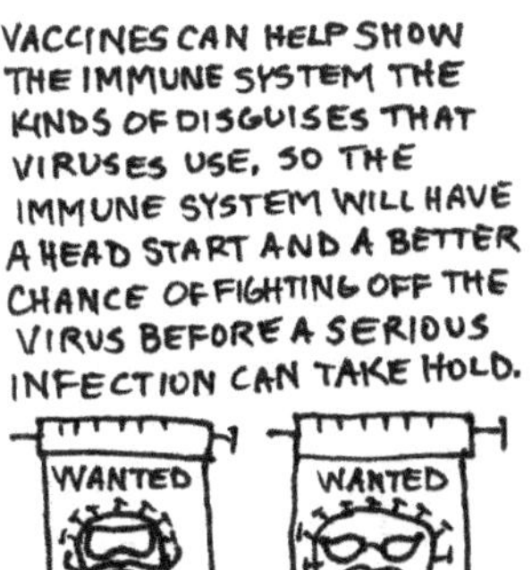

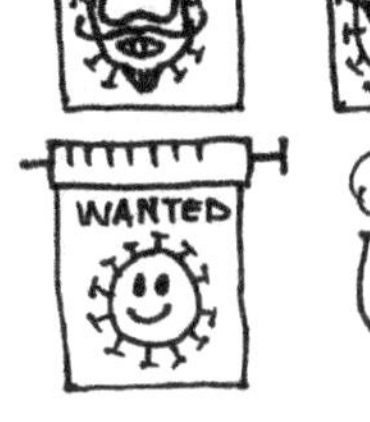

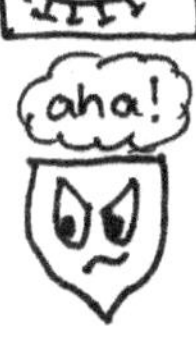

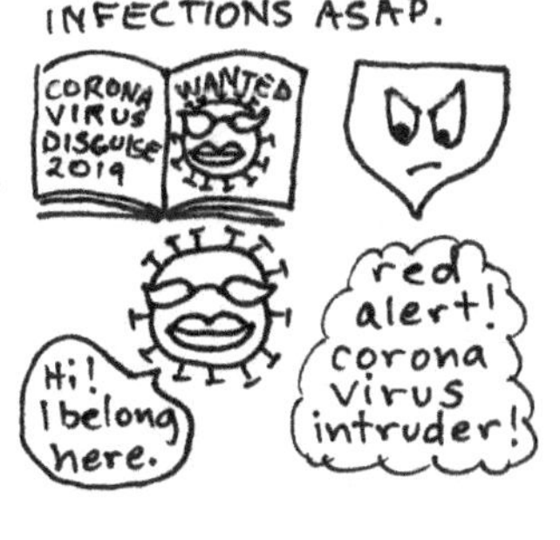

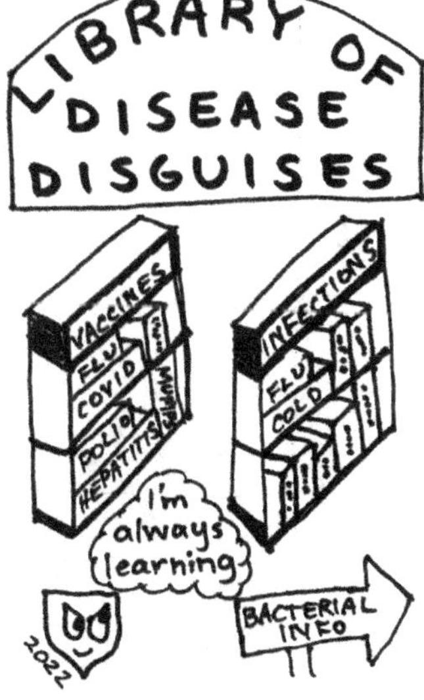

Art by Katie Bradshaw.

PANDEMIC
PANDEMIC
PANDEMIC
PANDEMIC VACCINATE
PANDEMIC VACCINATE
PANDEMIC VACCINATE
PANDEMIC VACCINATE

END THE PANDEMIC

GET VACCINATED

Art by Justin Kemerling.

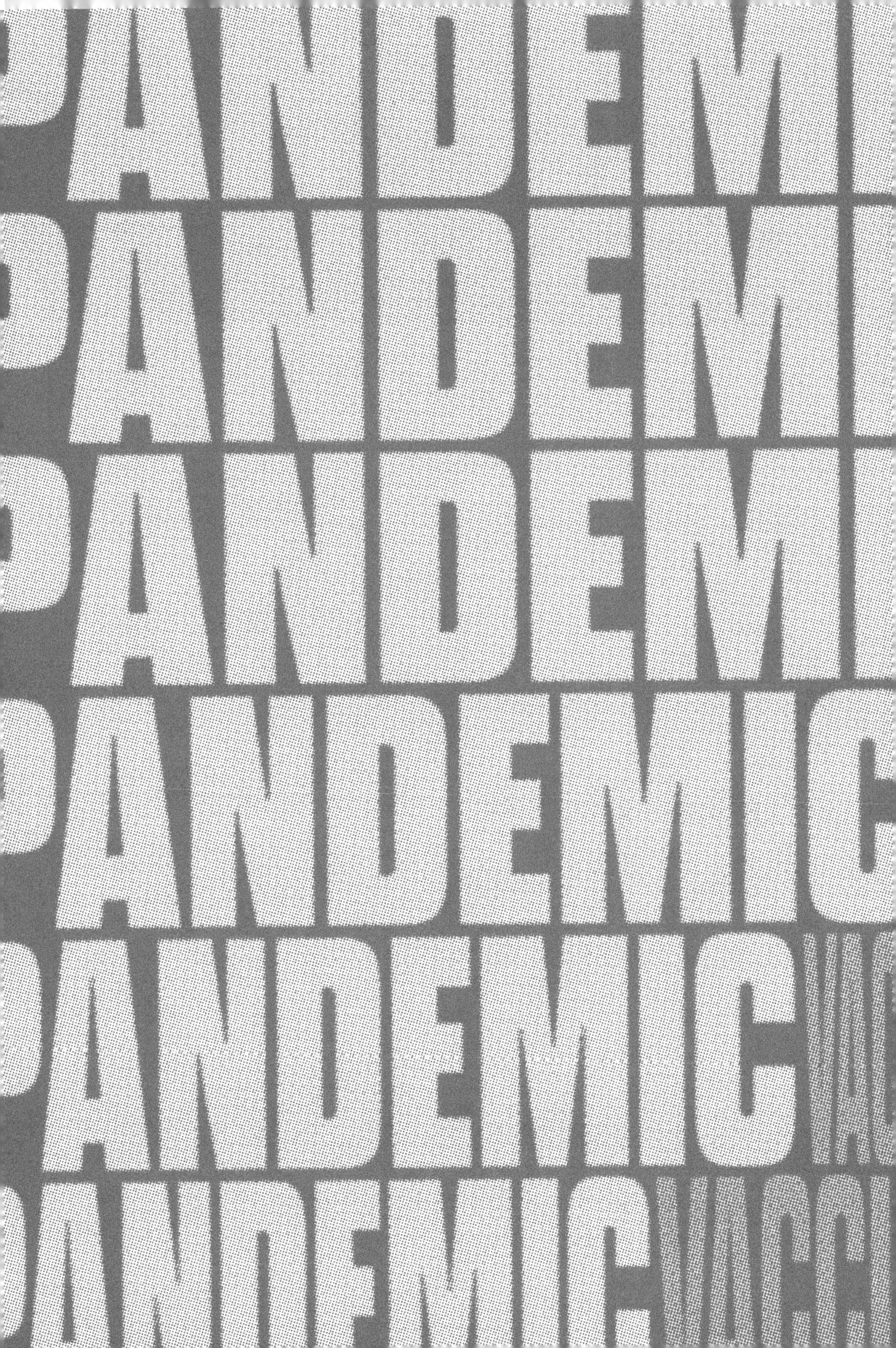

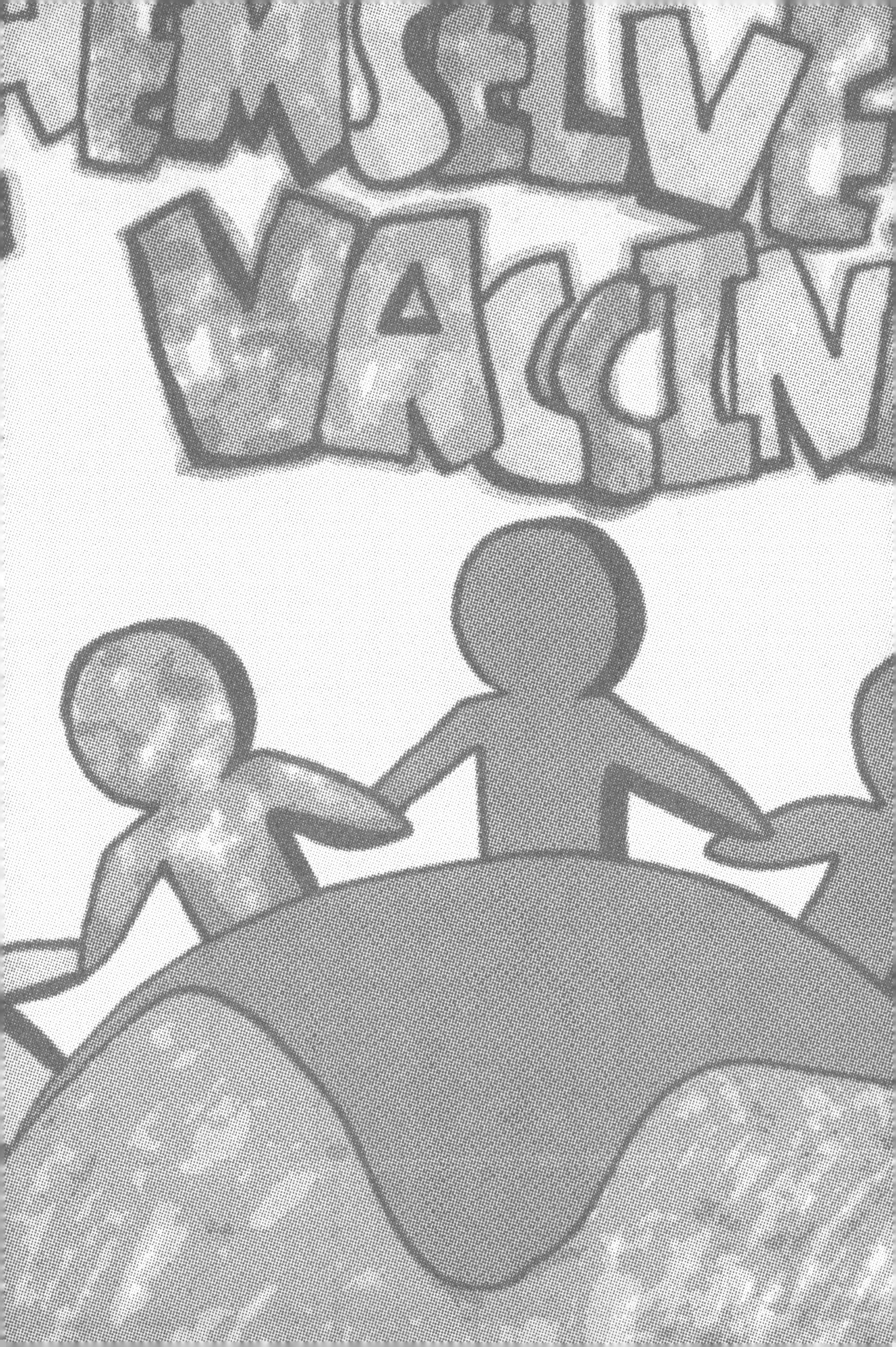

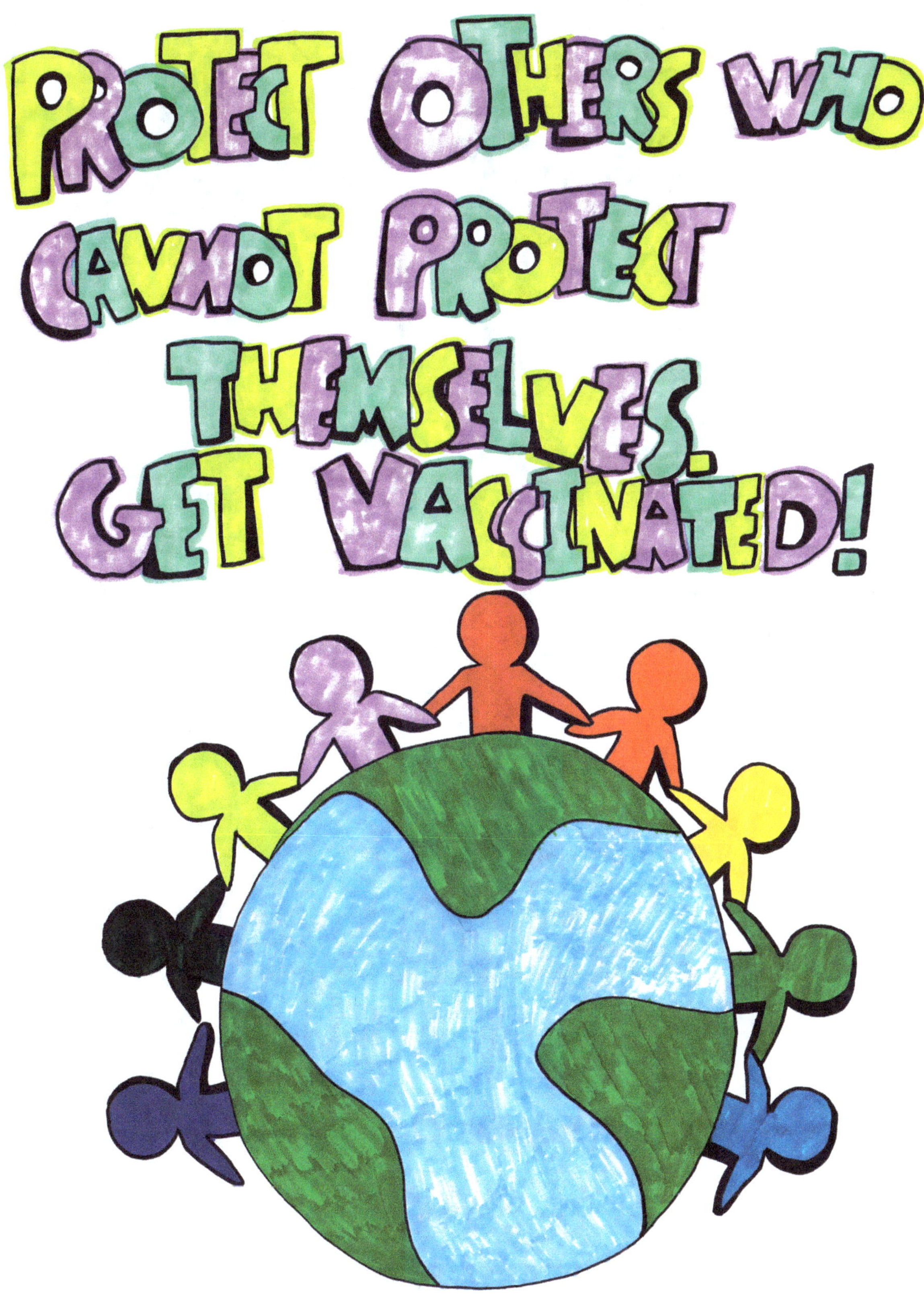

Art by Malia McCreight.

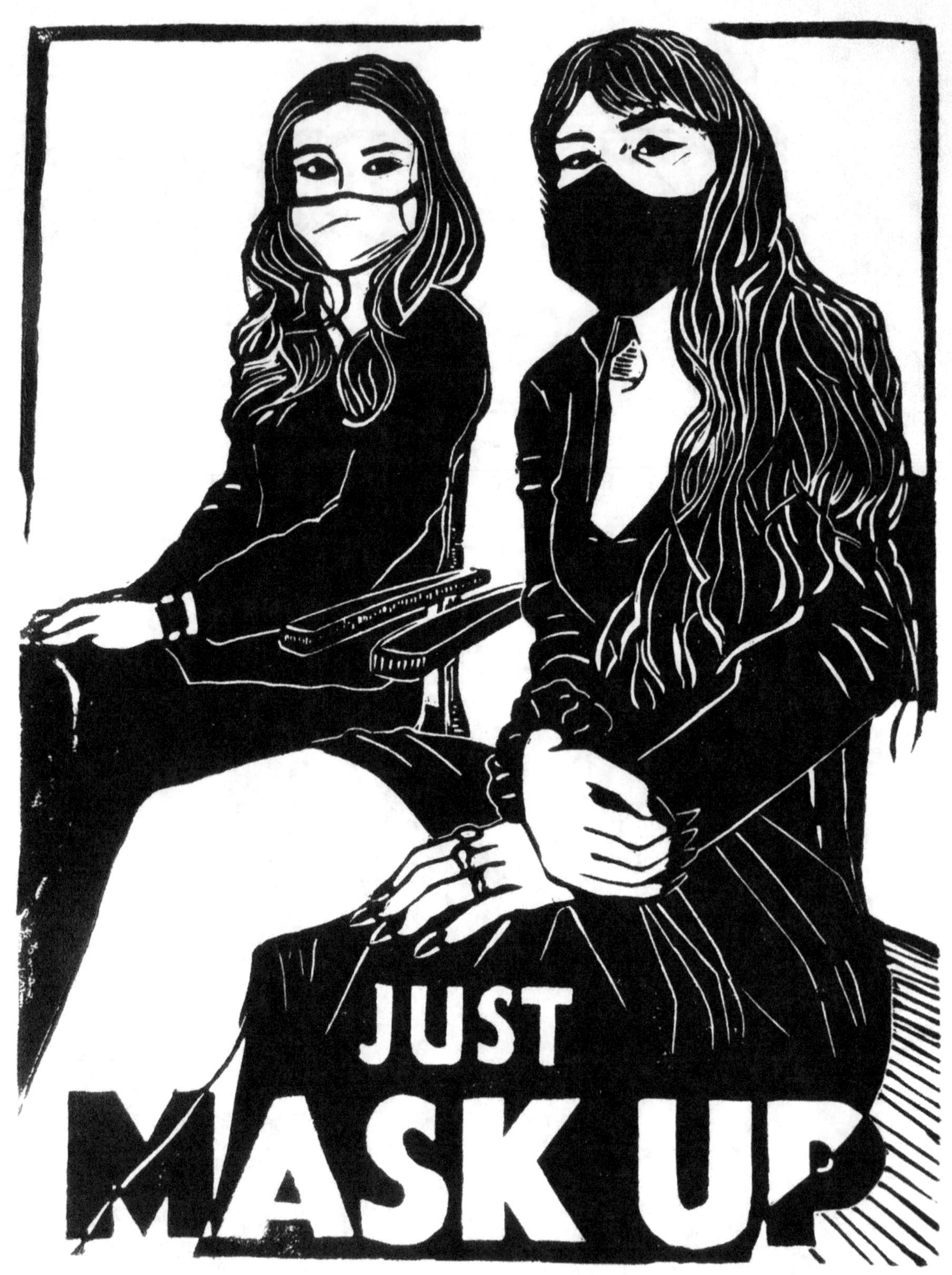

and
GET YOUR
COVID VACCINATIONS

Art by Ben Darling.

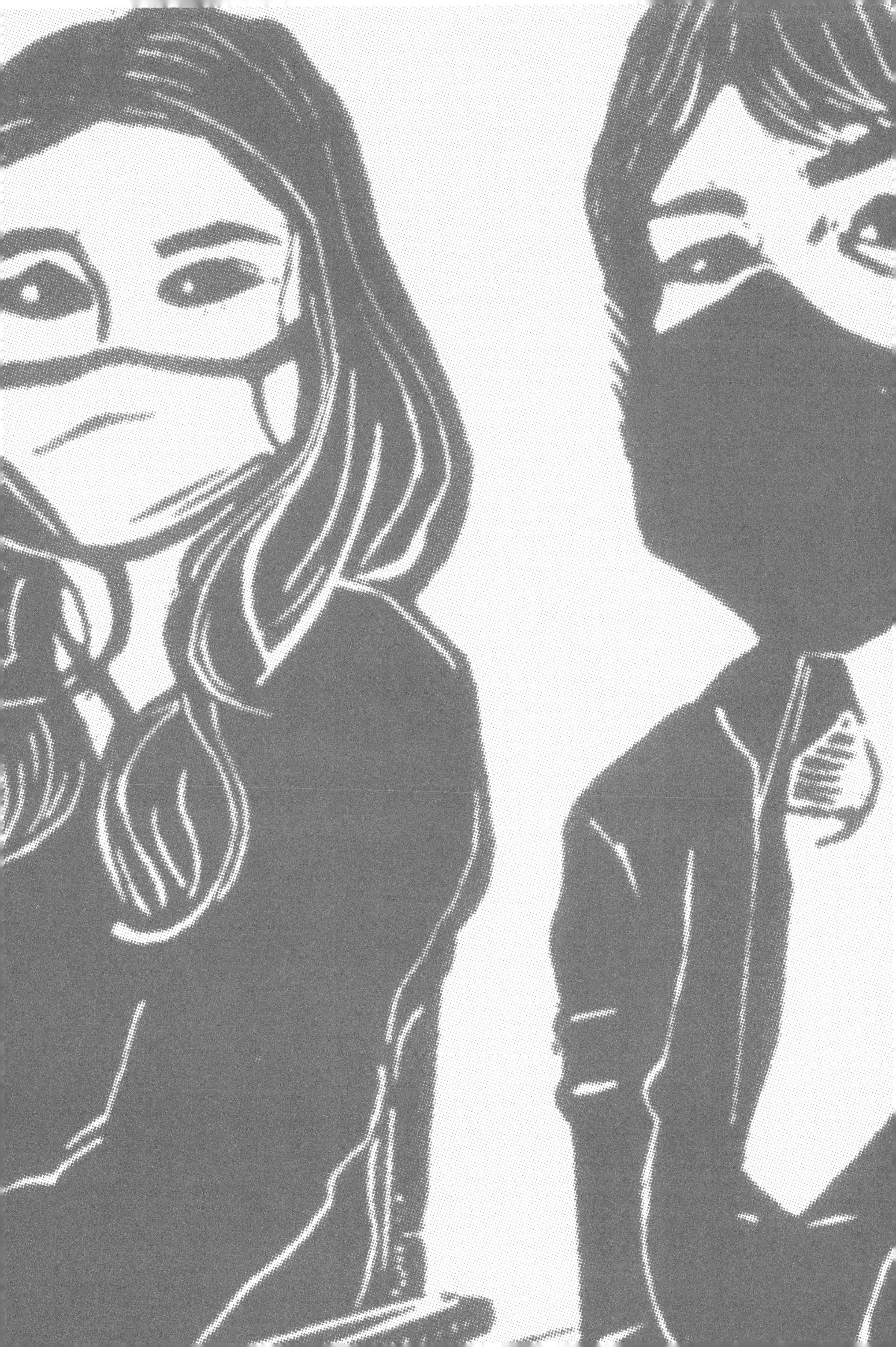

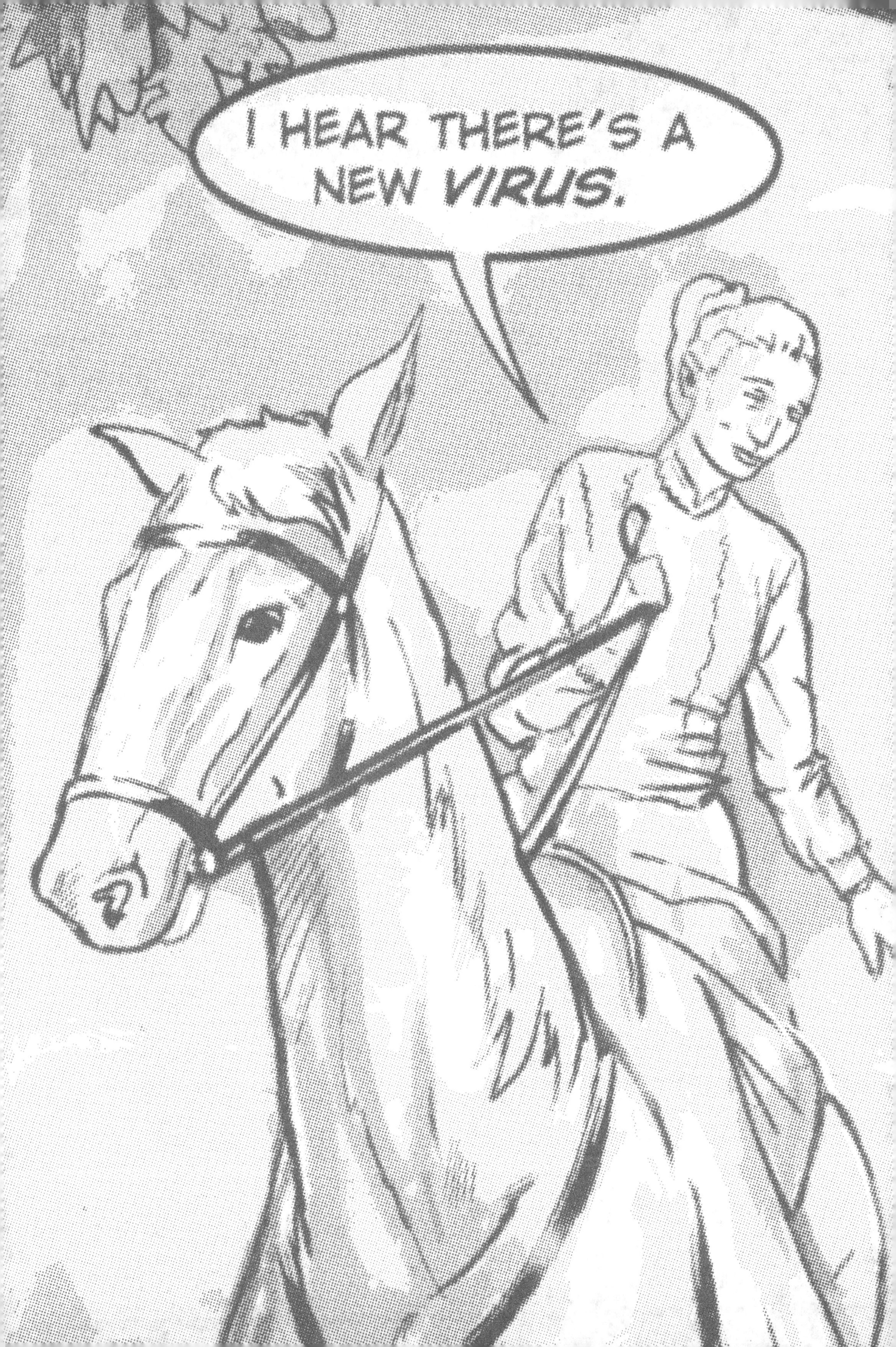
I HEAR THERE'S A NEW VIRUS.

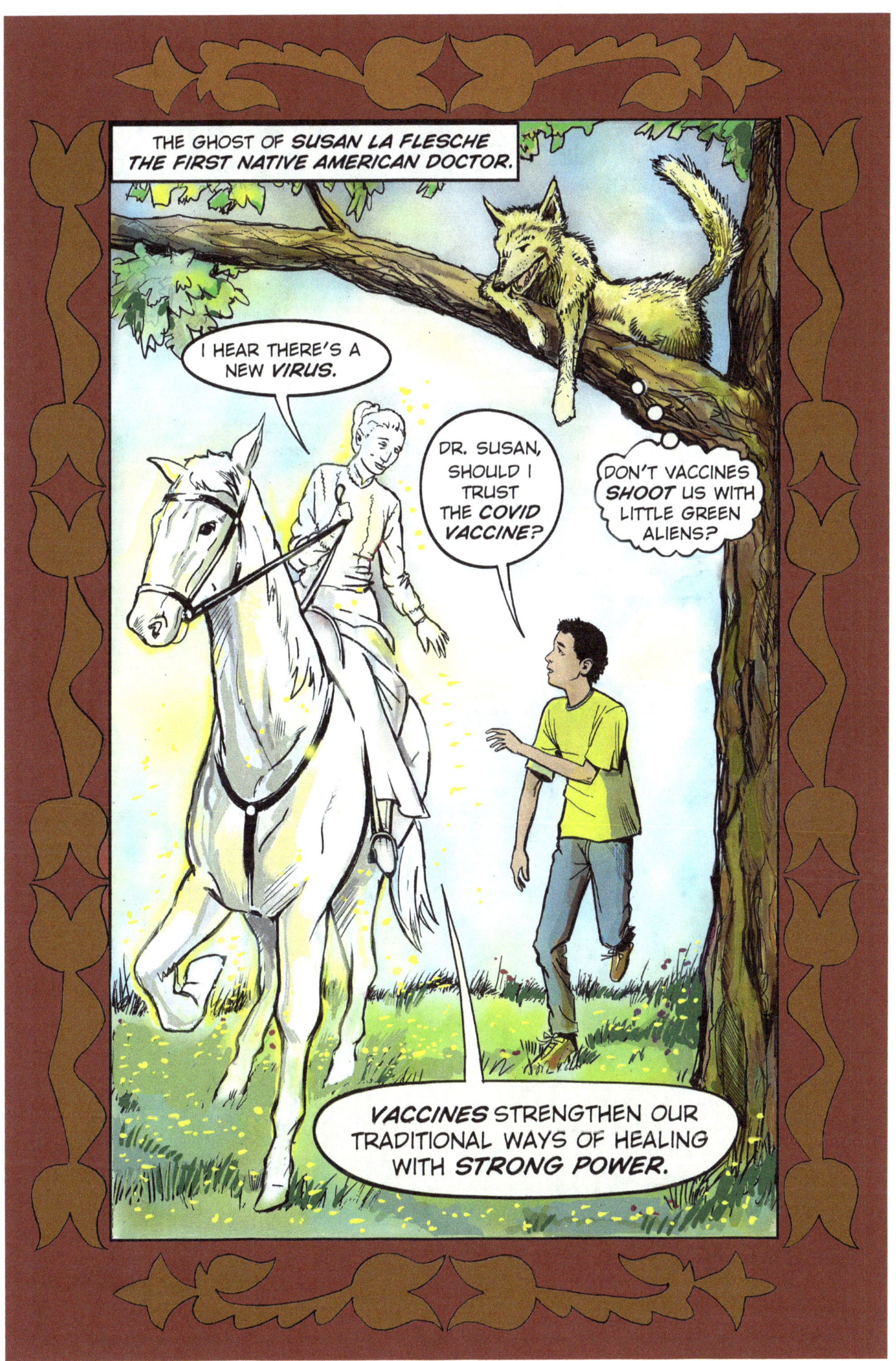

Art by Henry Payer and Bob Hall.

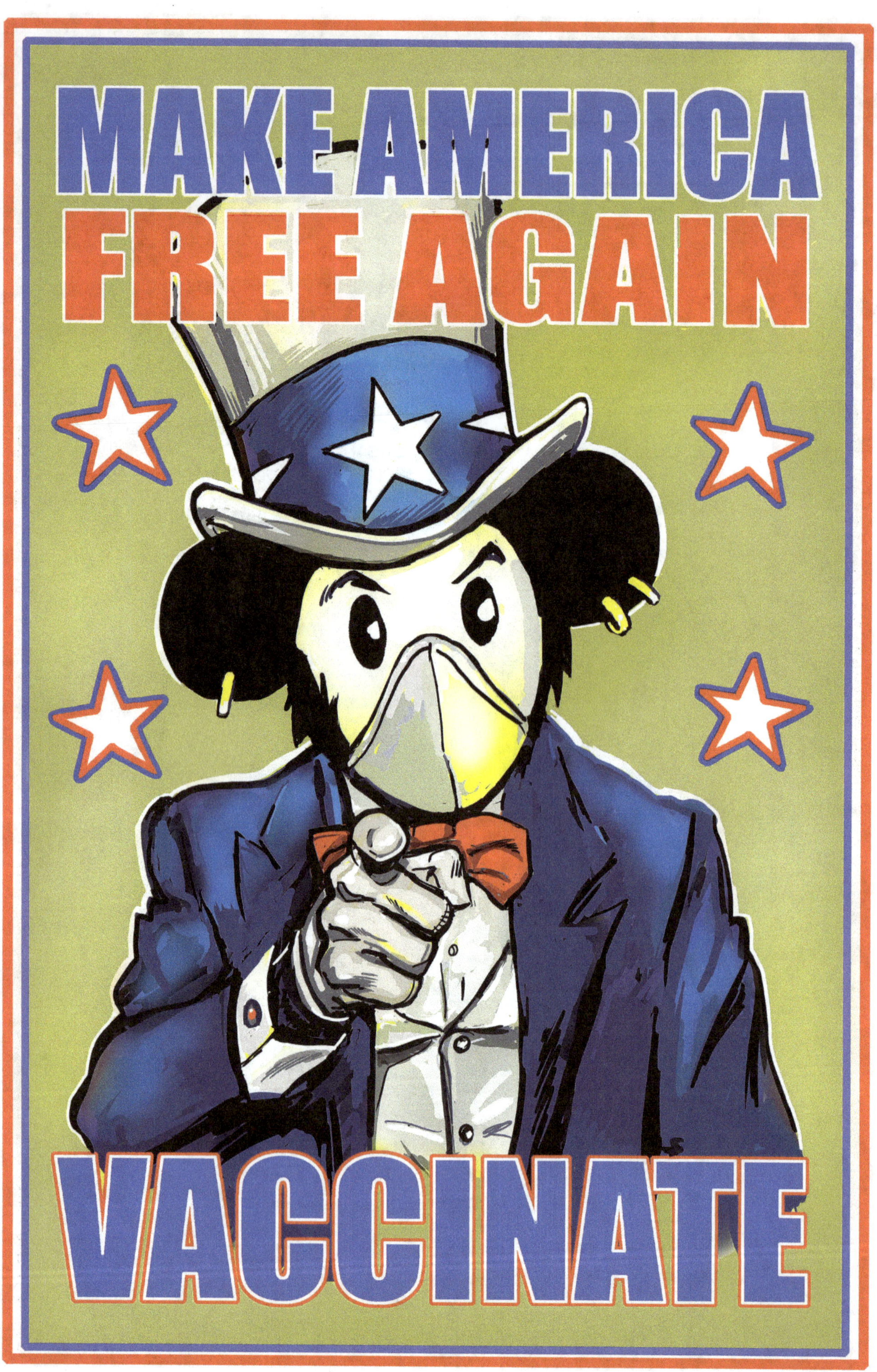

Art by Bob Hall.

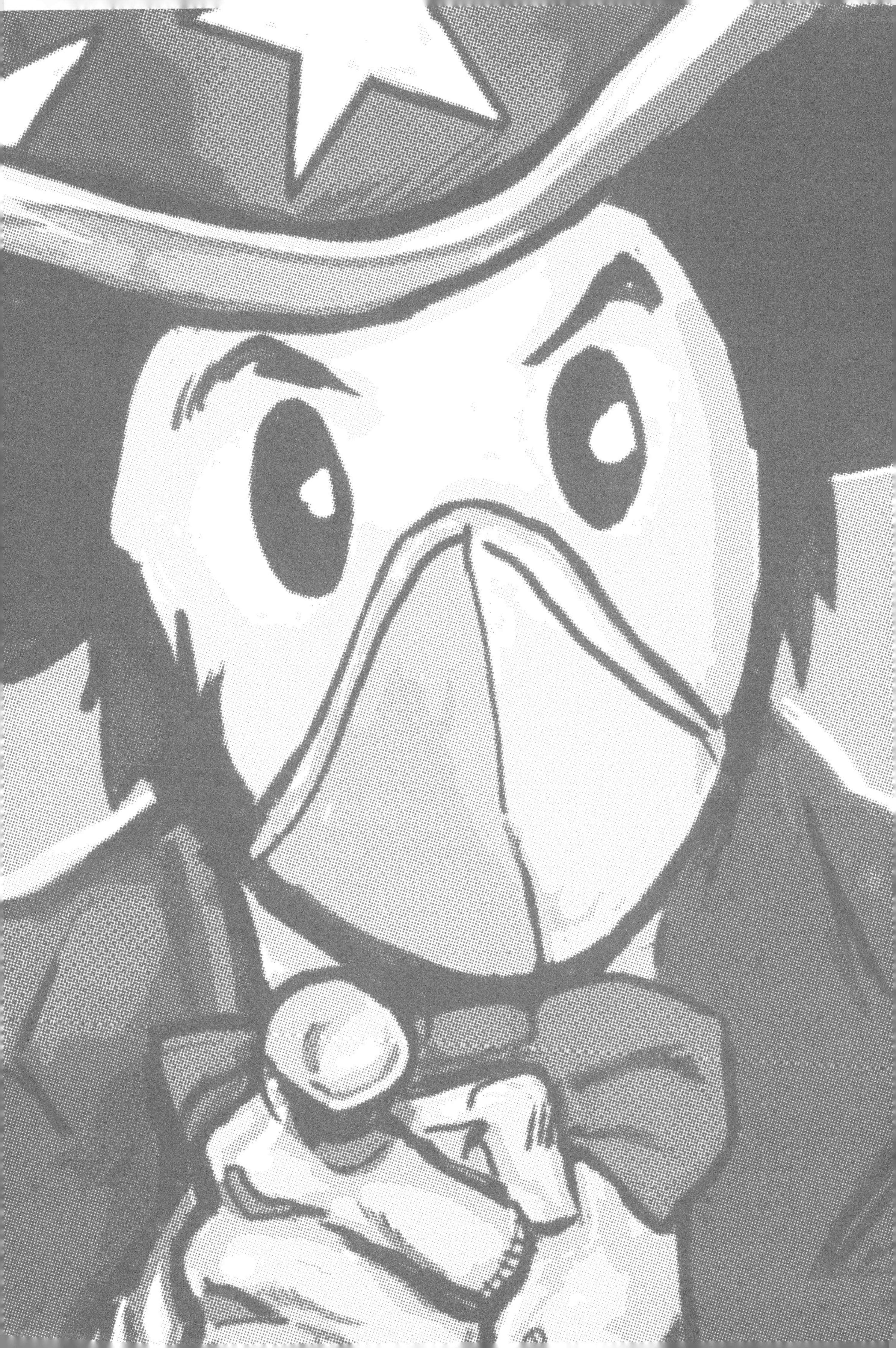

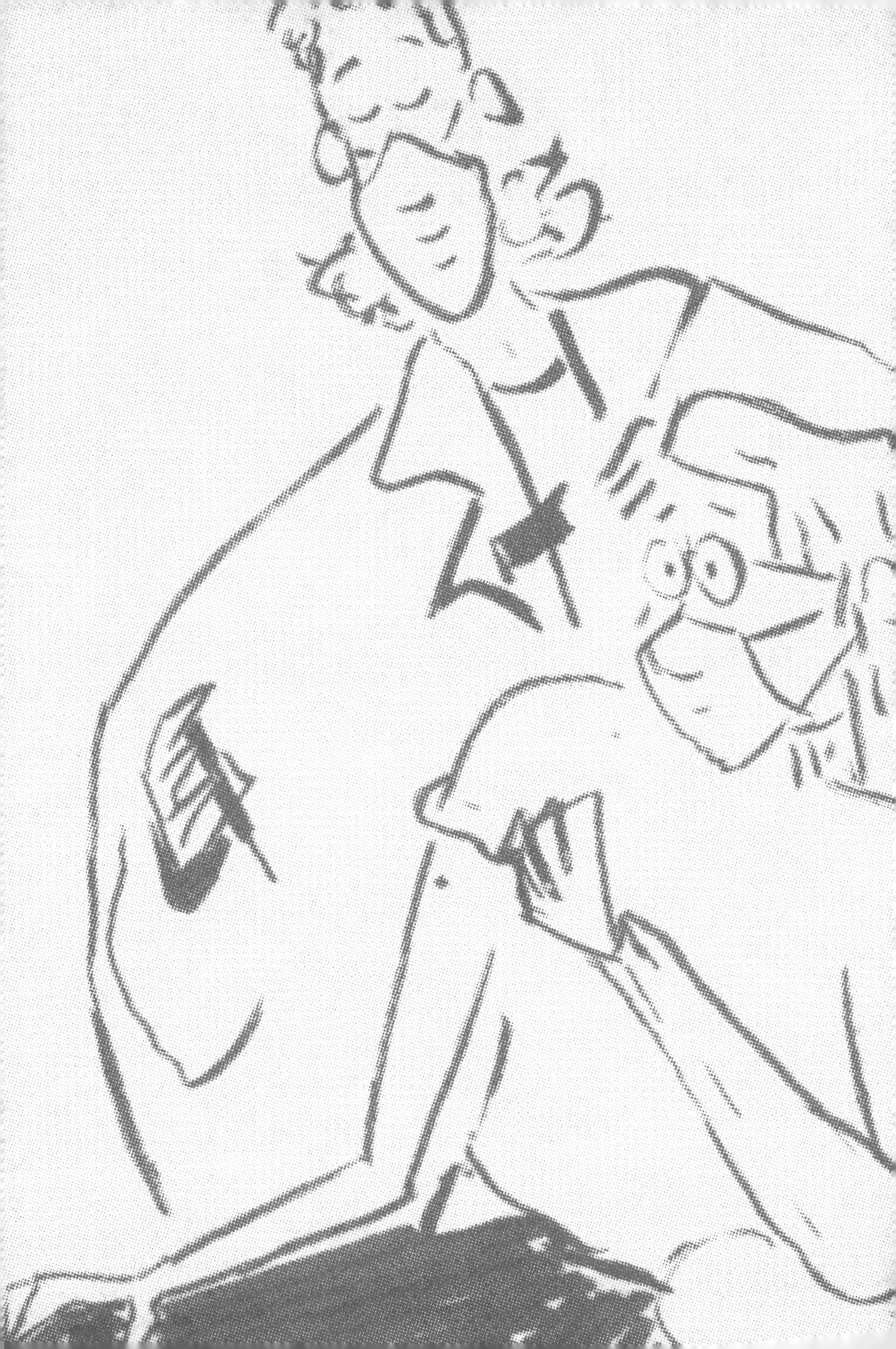

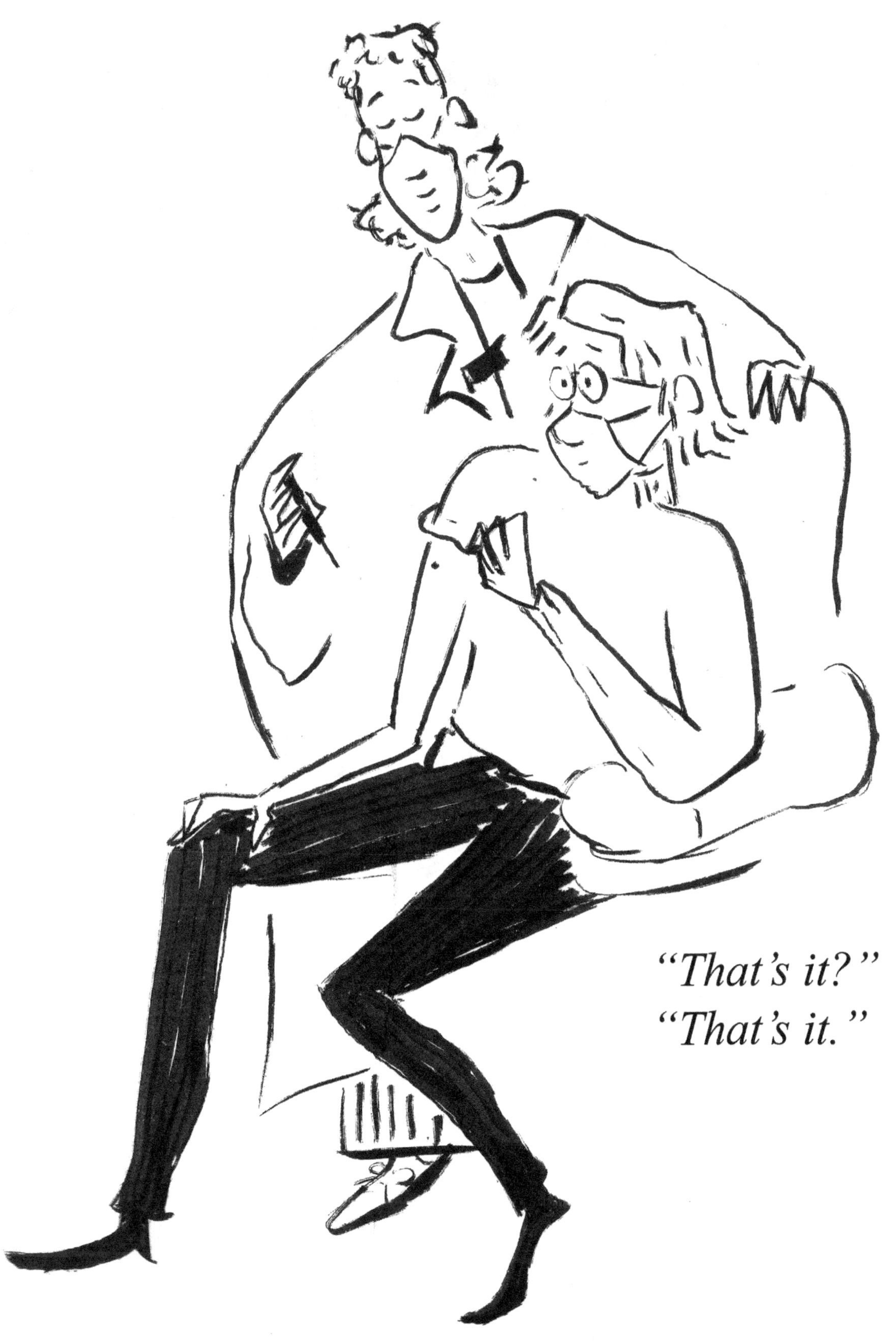

"That's it?"
"That's it."

Art by Eric Morris.

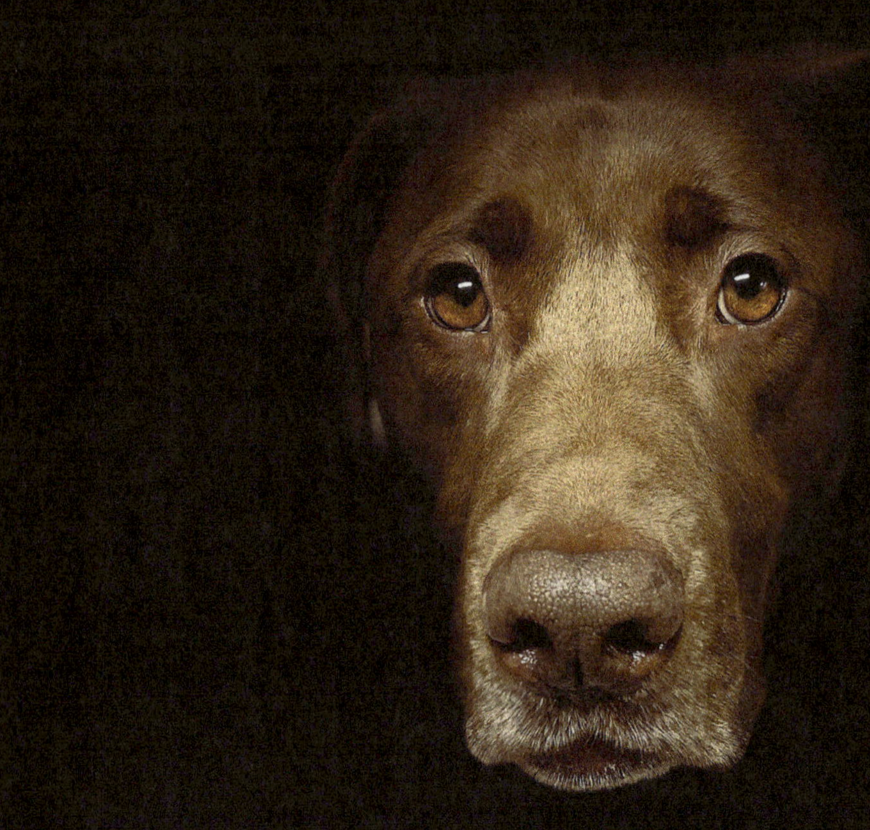

I AM WORRIED ABOUT MY HUMANS!

VACCINATE TODAY

Art by Janet Walters. Photography by Benjamin Walters.

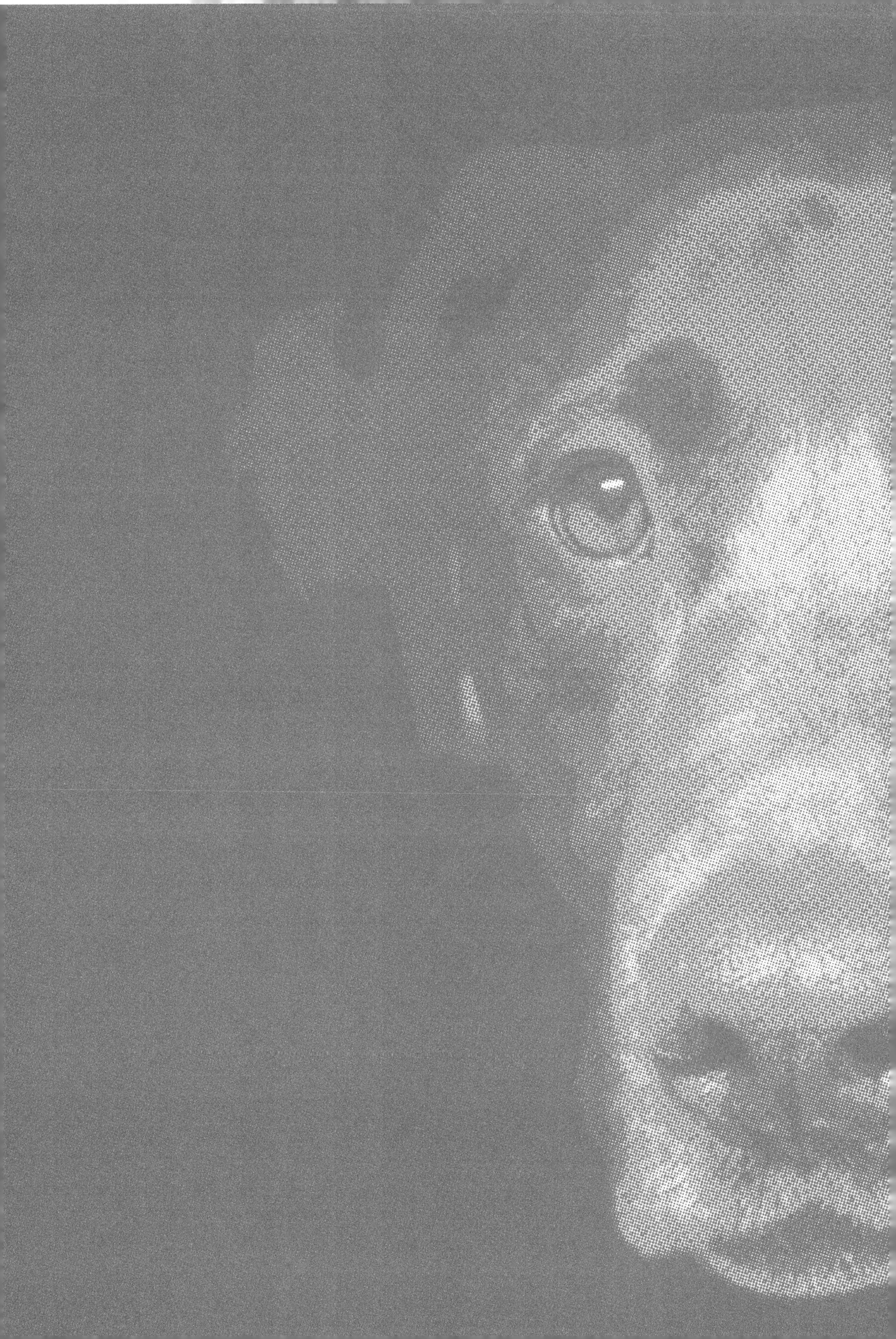

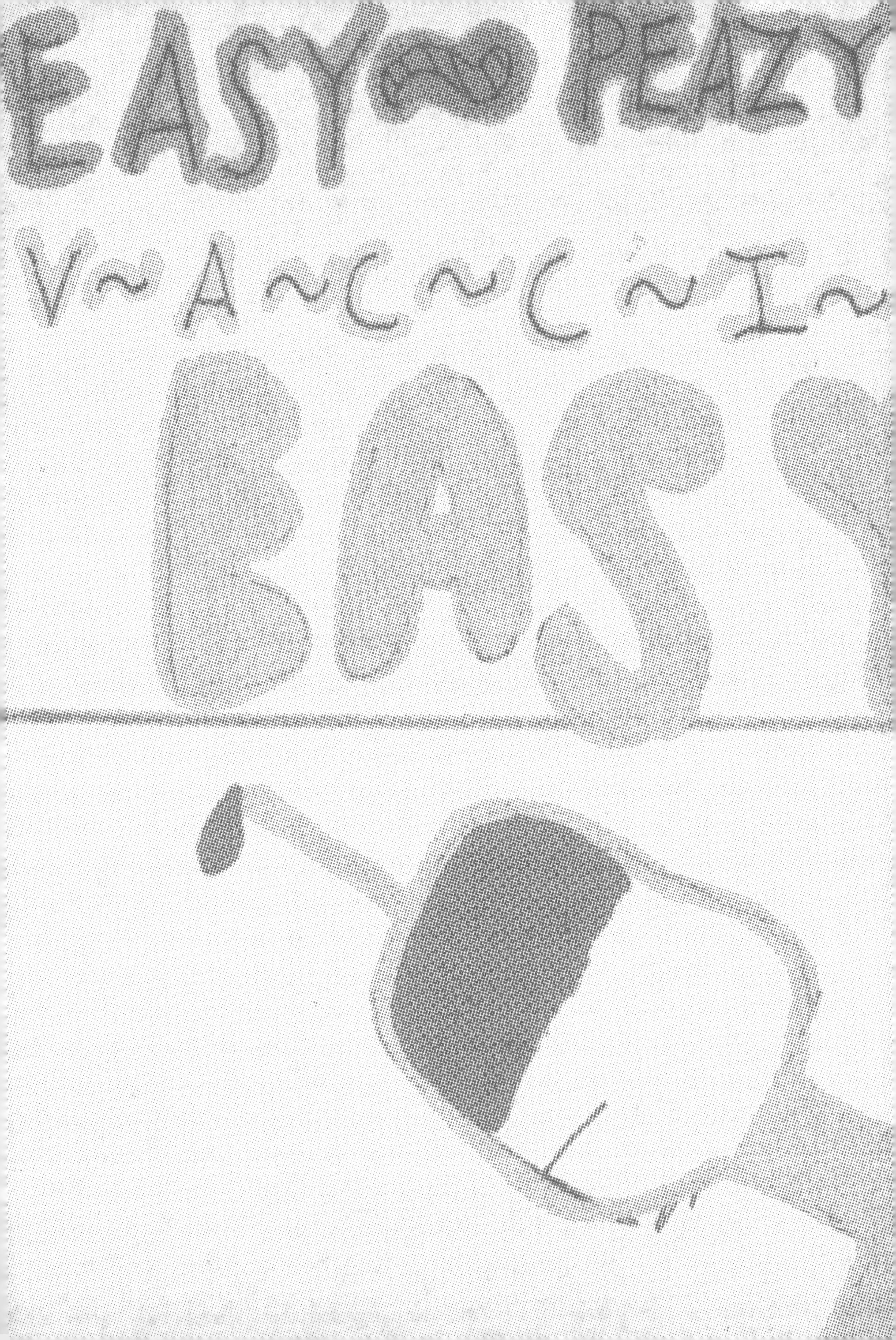
EASY PEAZY
V~A~C~C~I~
BAS

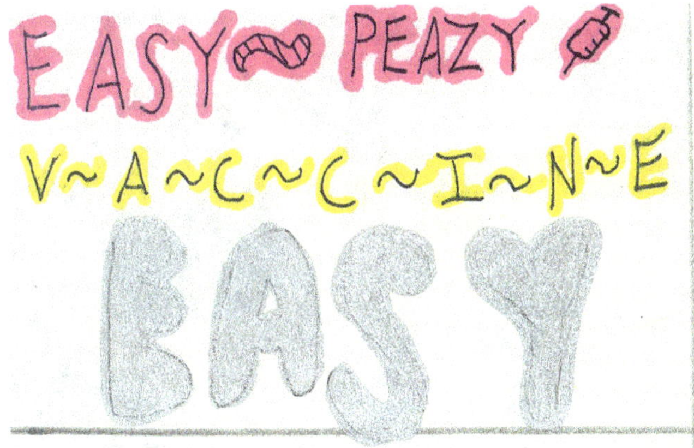

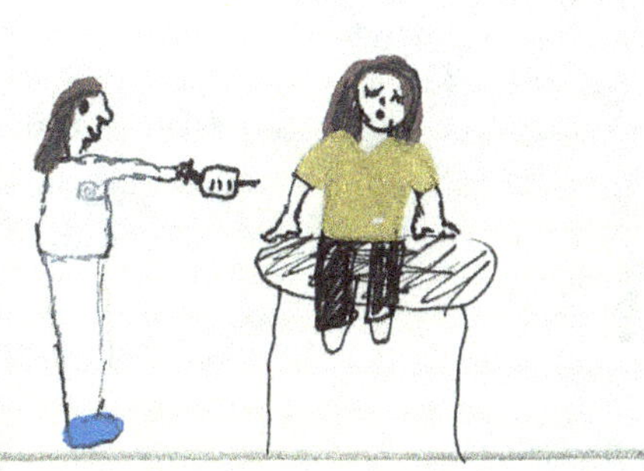

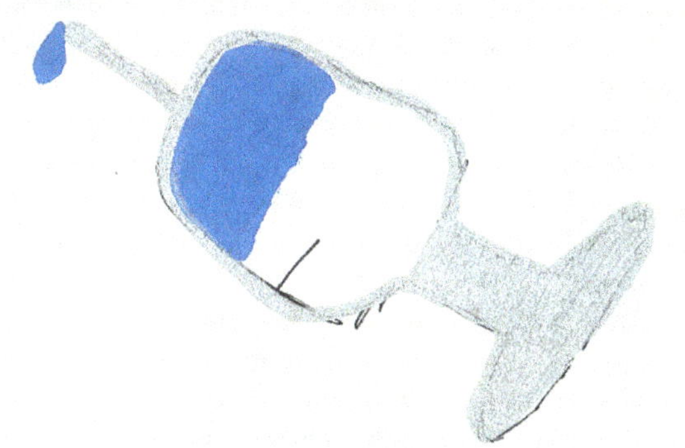

Keep calm and vaccine on

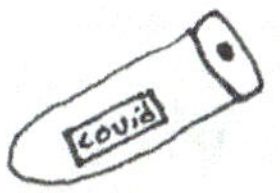

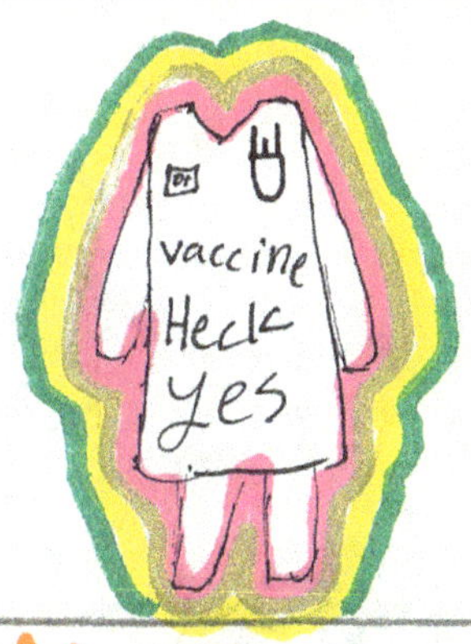

Scientists worked hard To find the vaccine so thank them by using it.

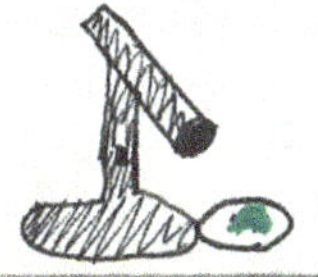

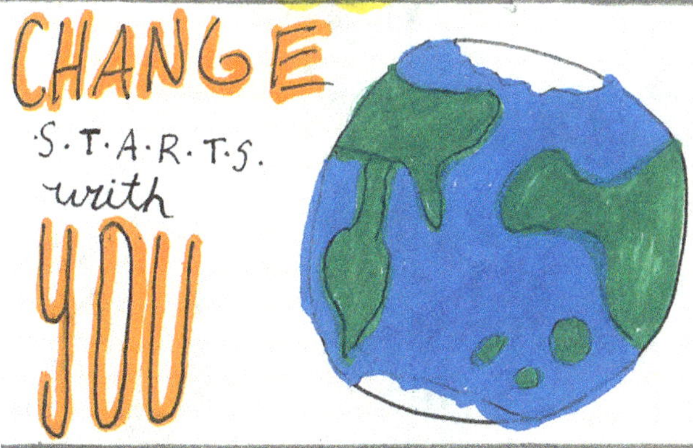

USE IT DONT ·L·O·S·E· IT

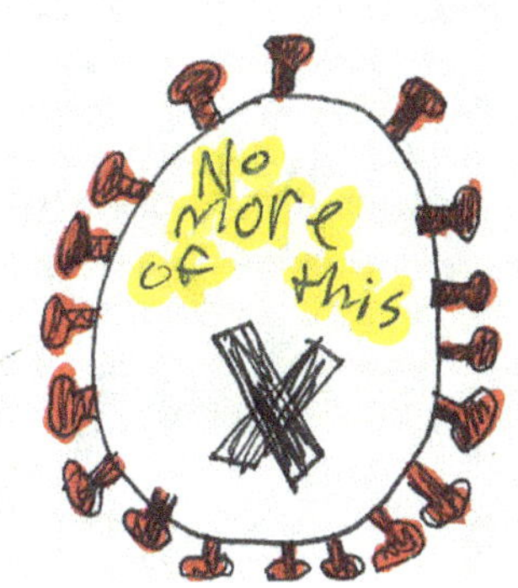

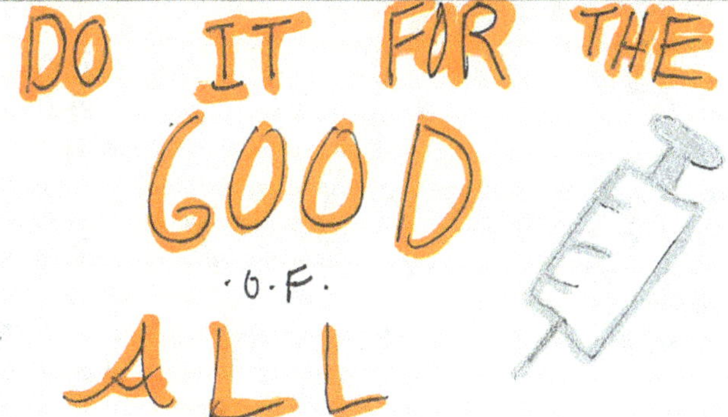

Art by Natalie Pulte.

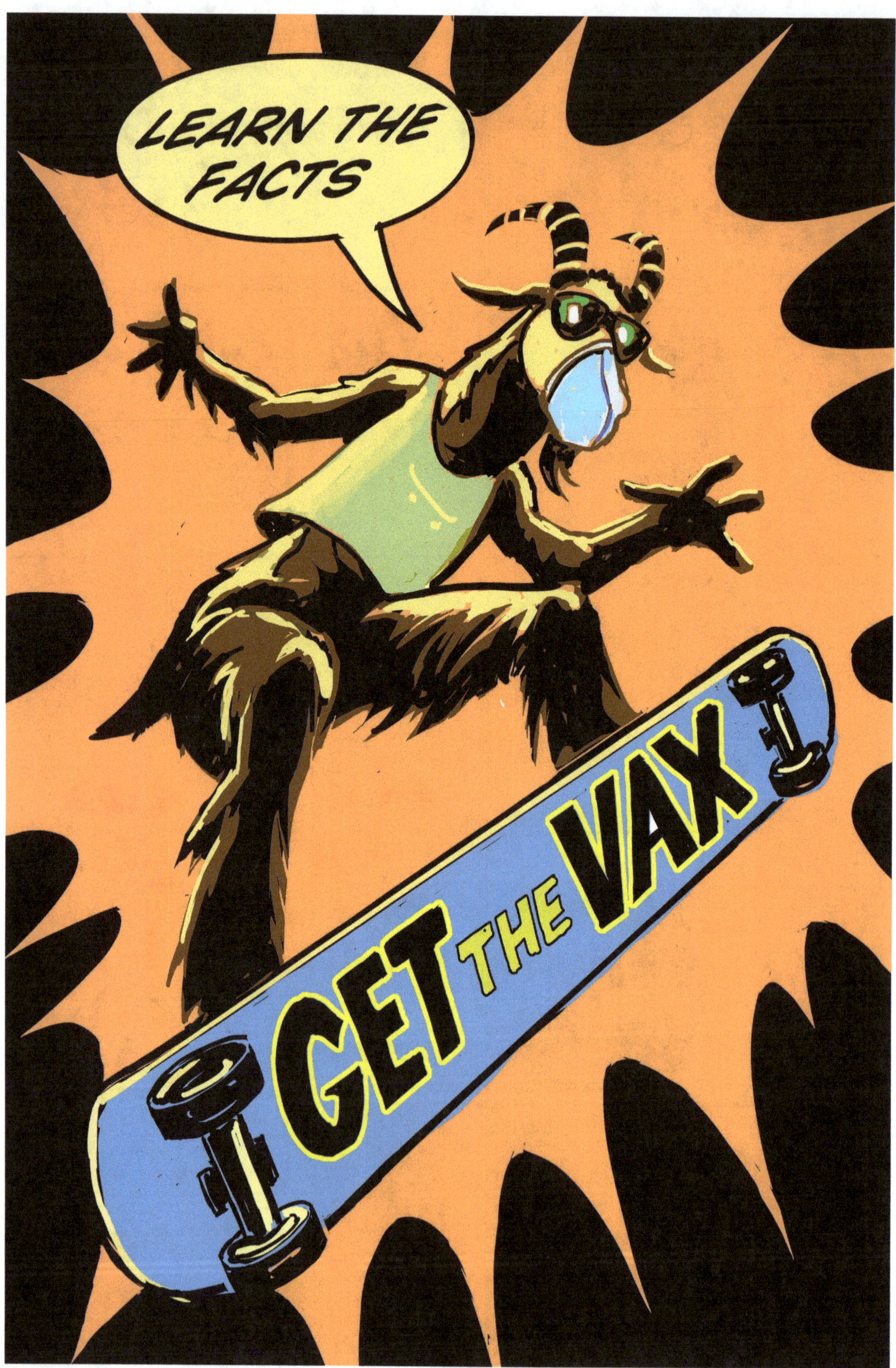

Art by Bob Hall.

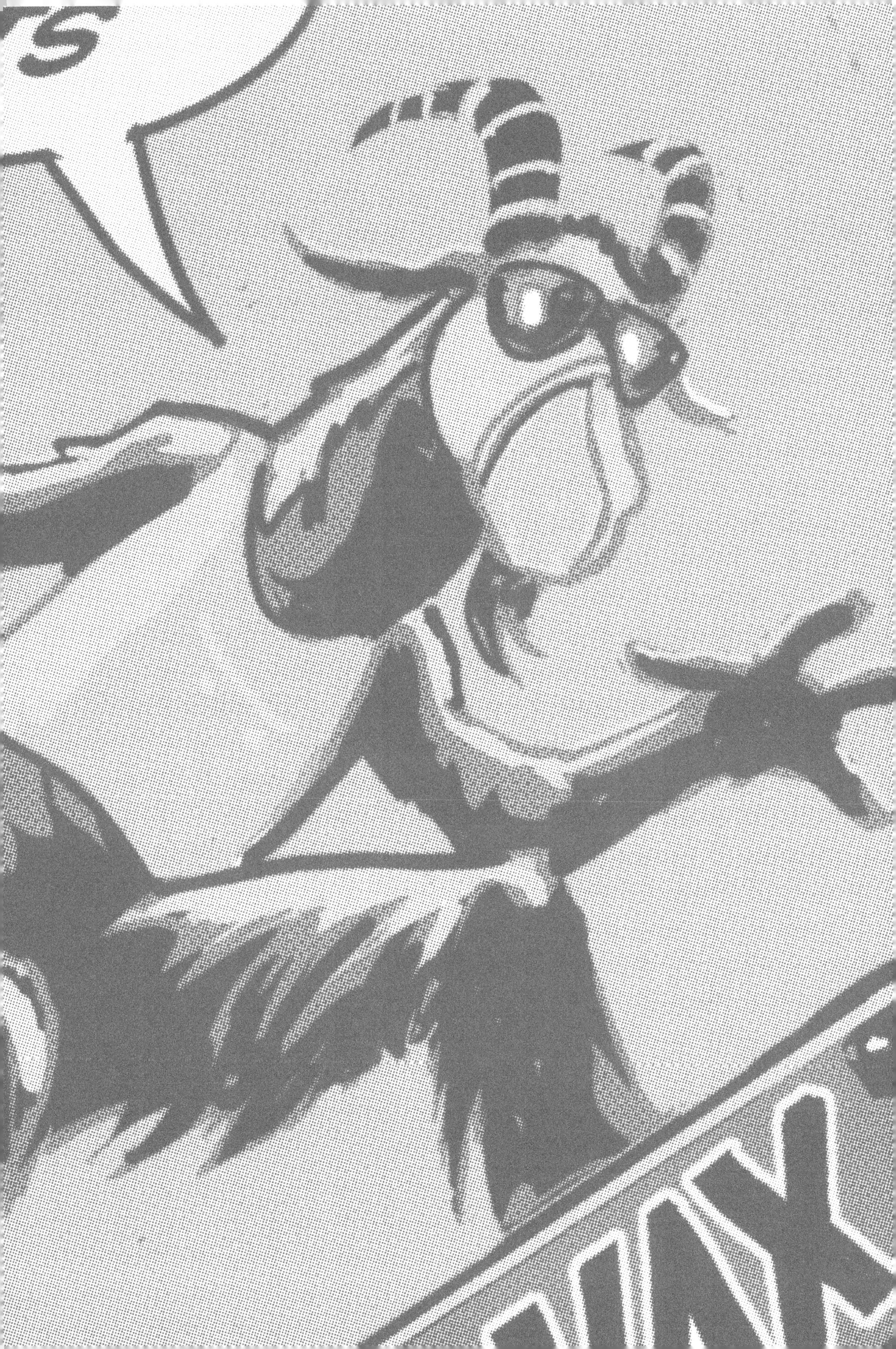

My parents said that I didn't have to get vaccinated.

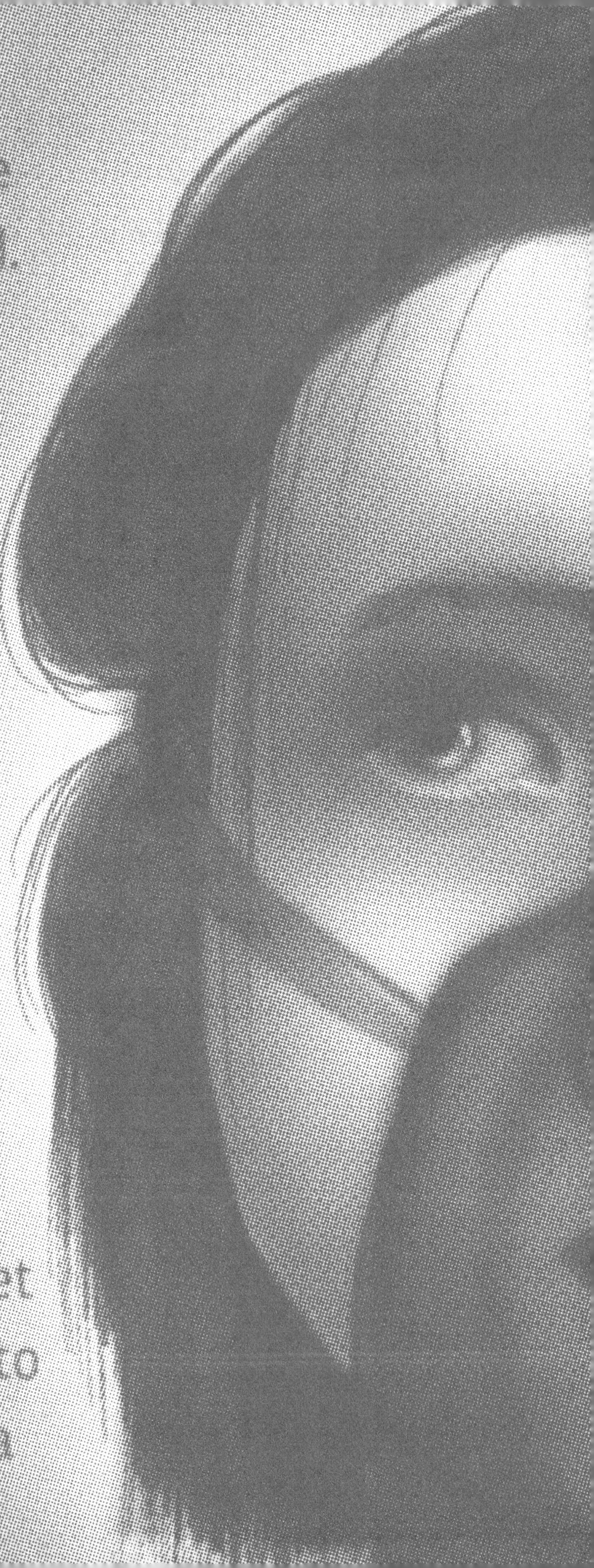

They said kids my age didn't die.

It's sad I only get to say goodbye to them through a glass window.

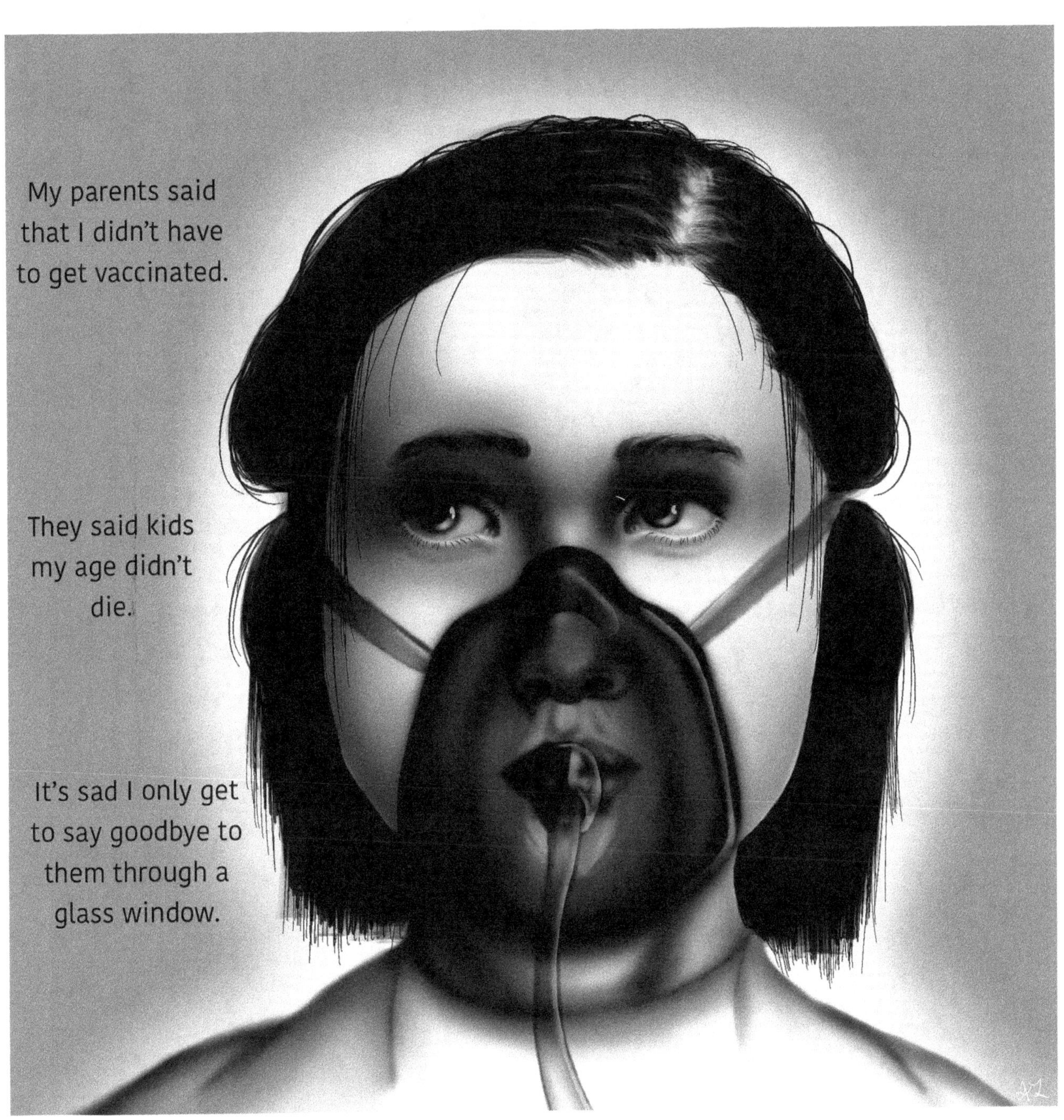

Art by Anna Lindstrom.

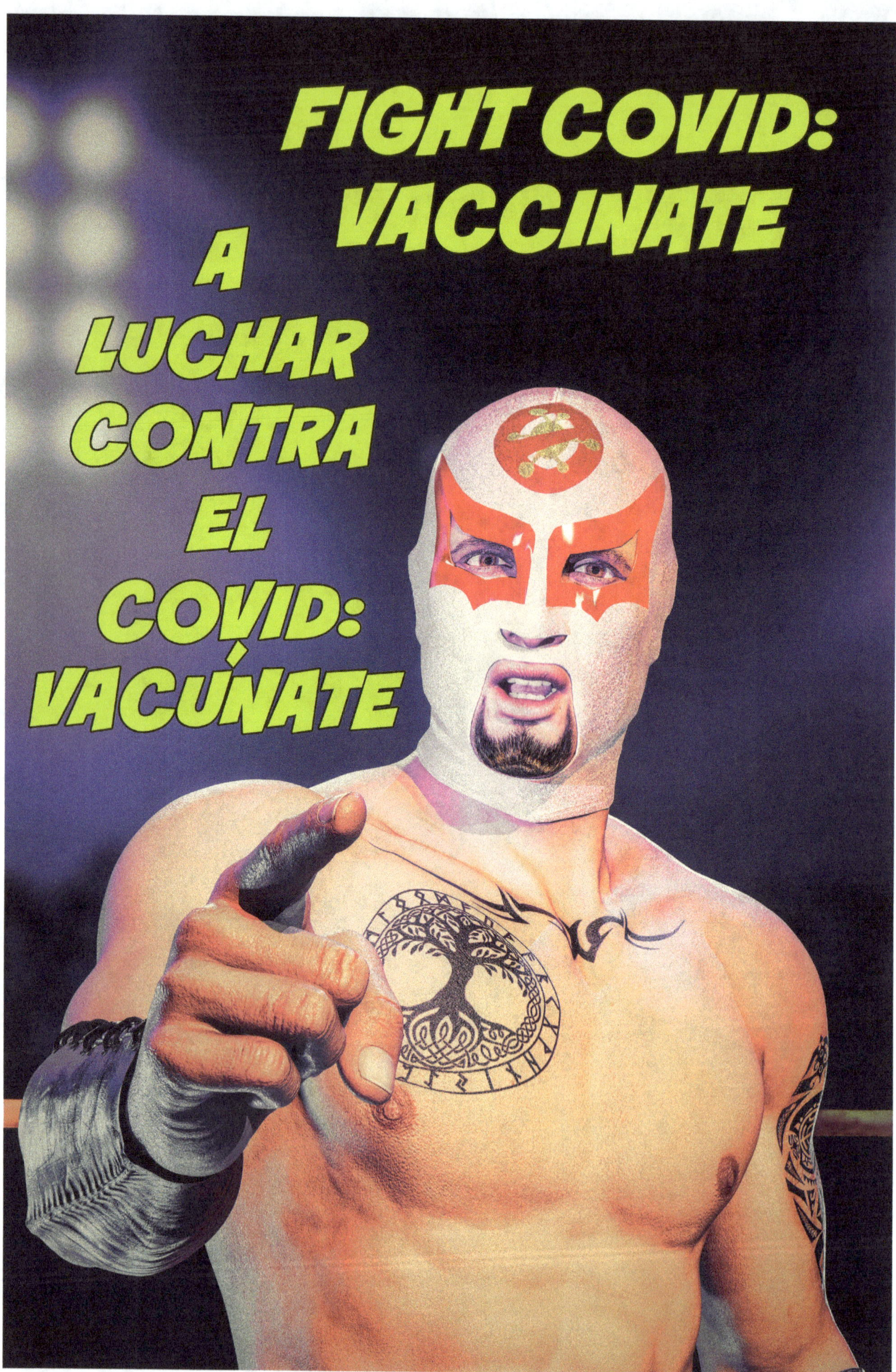

Art by Heinzy Cruz.

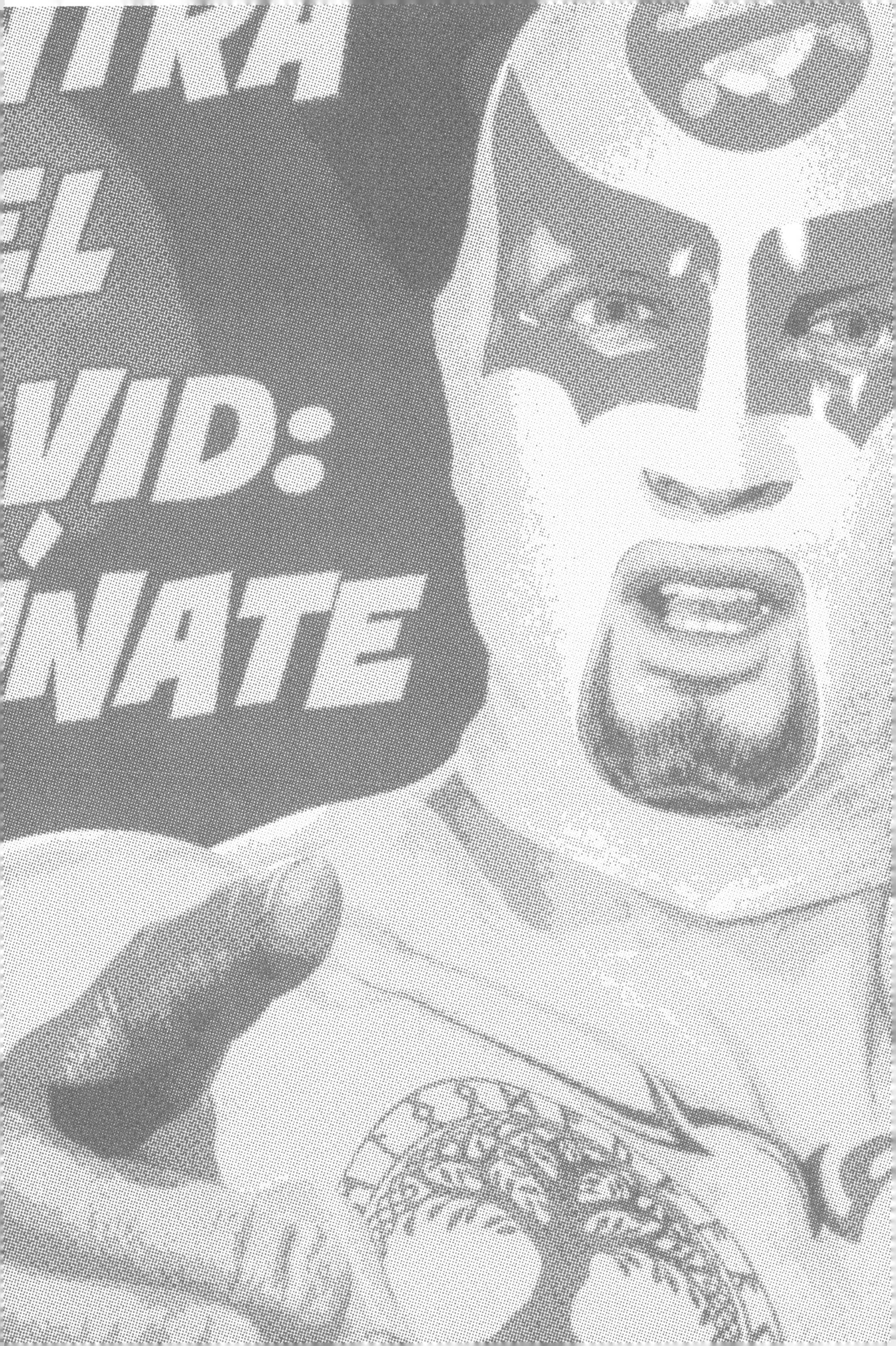

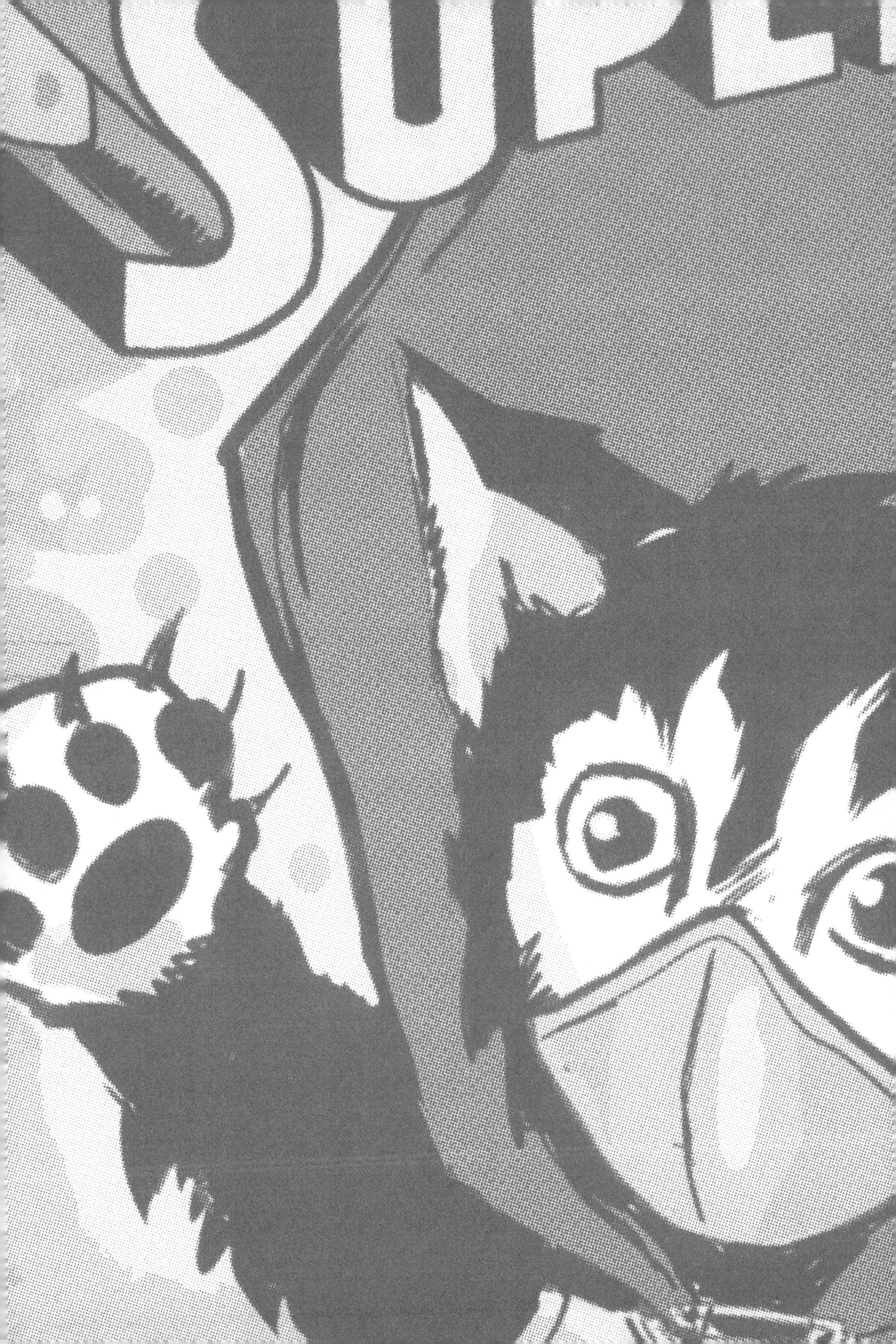

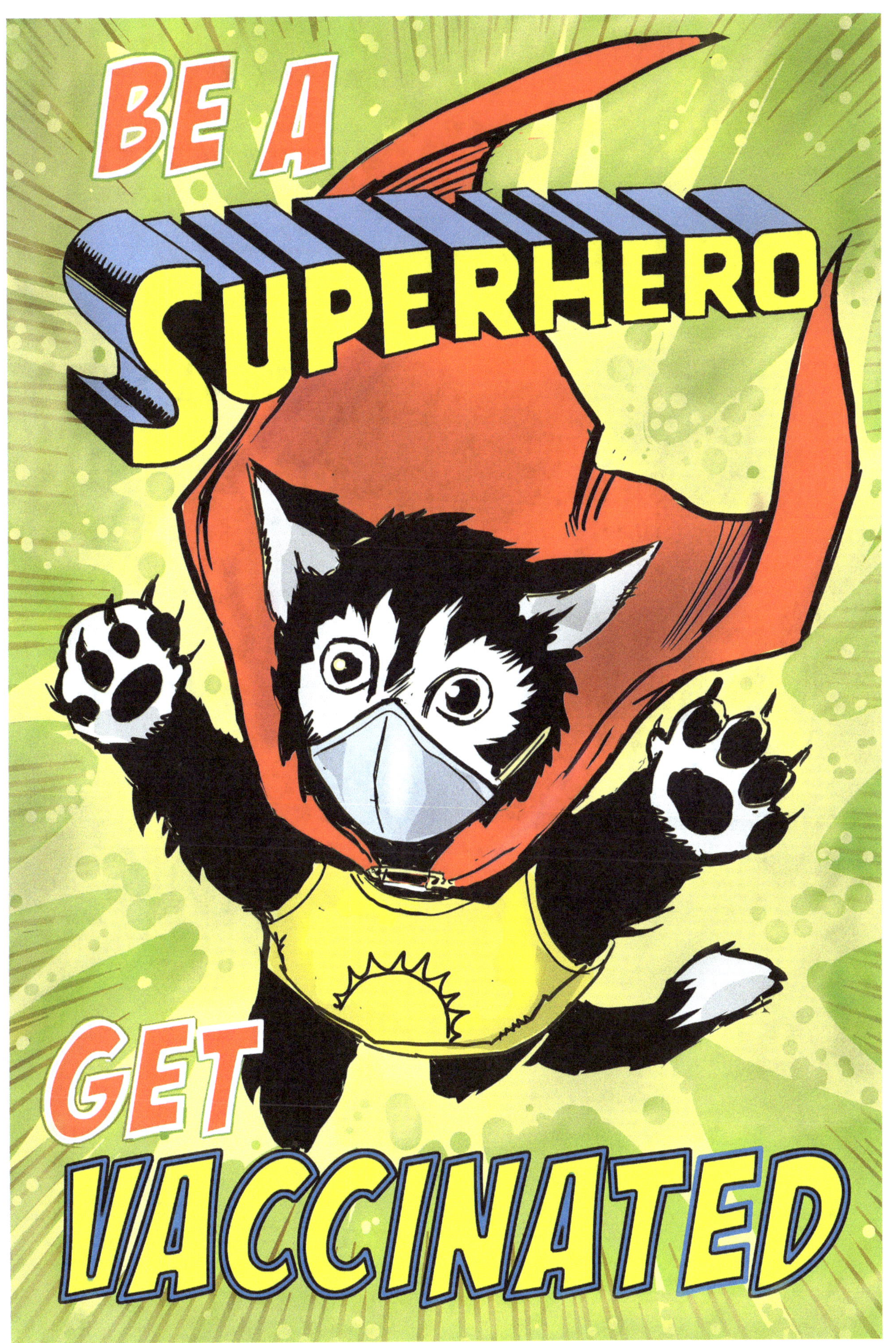

Art by Bob Hall.

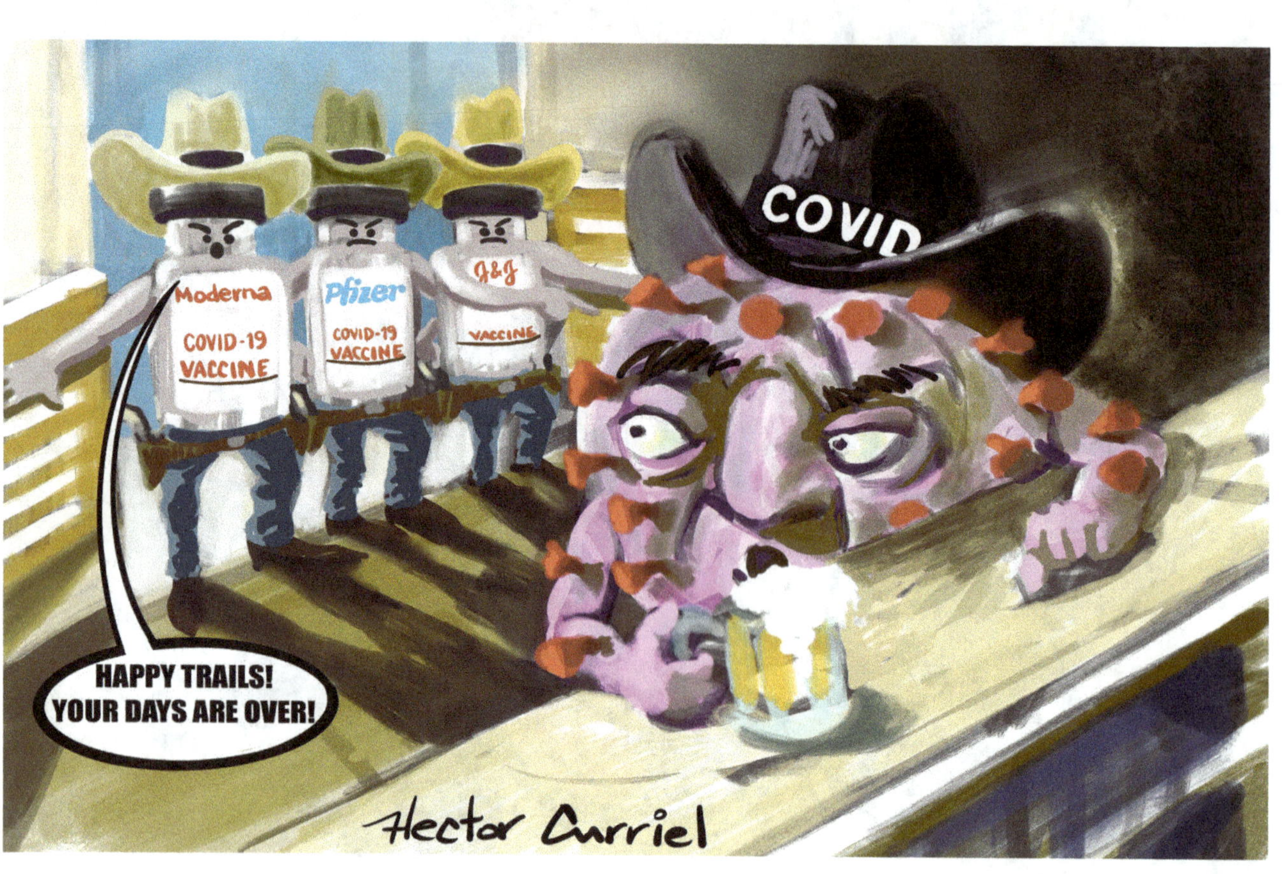

Art by Hector Curriel.

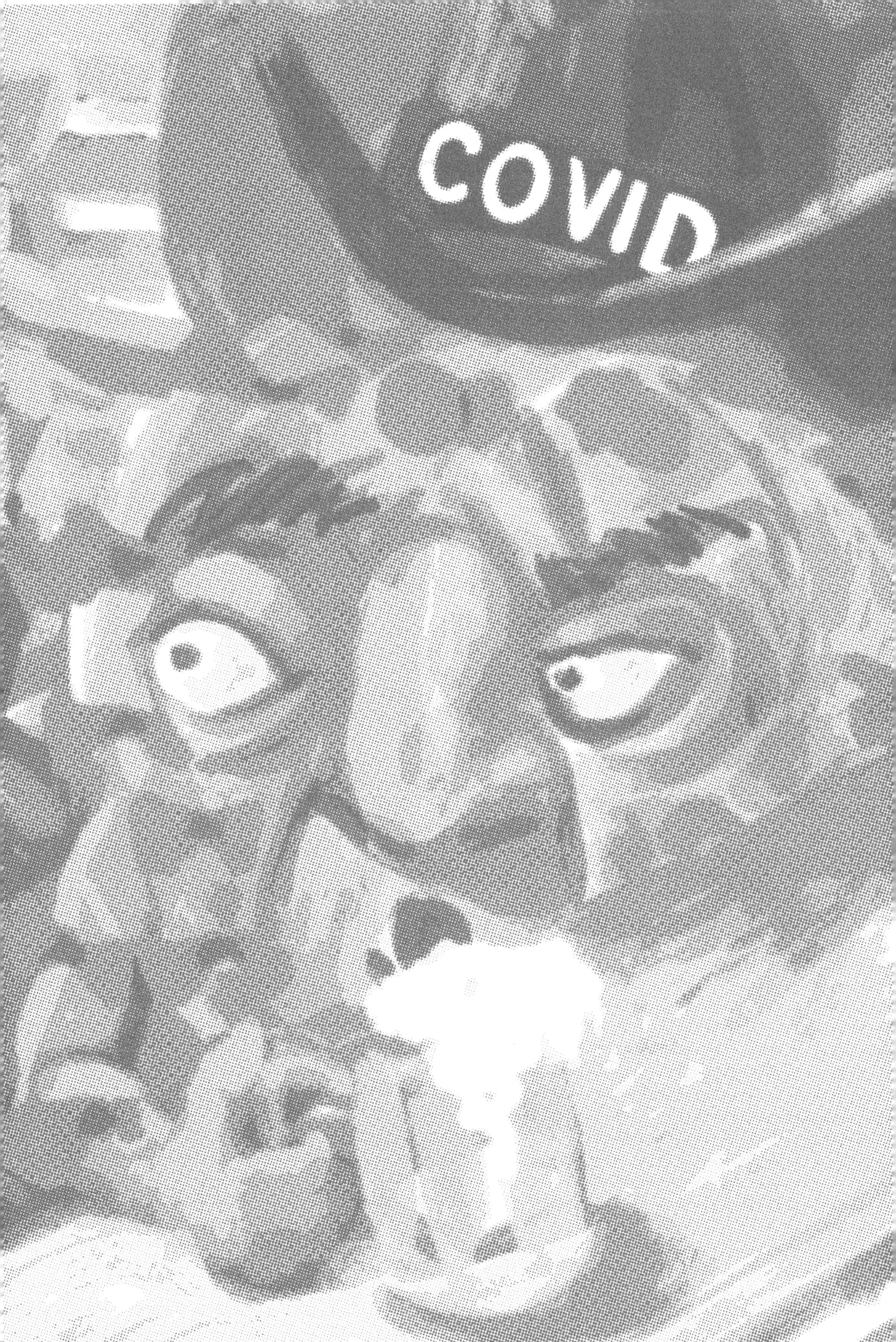
COVID

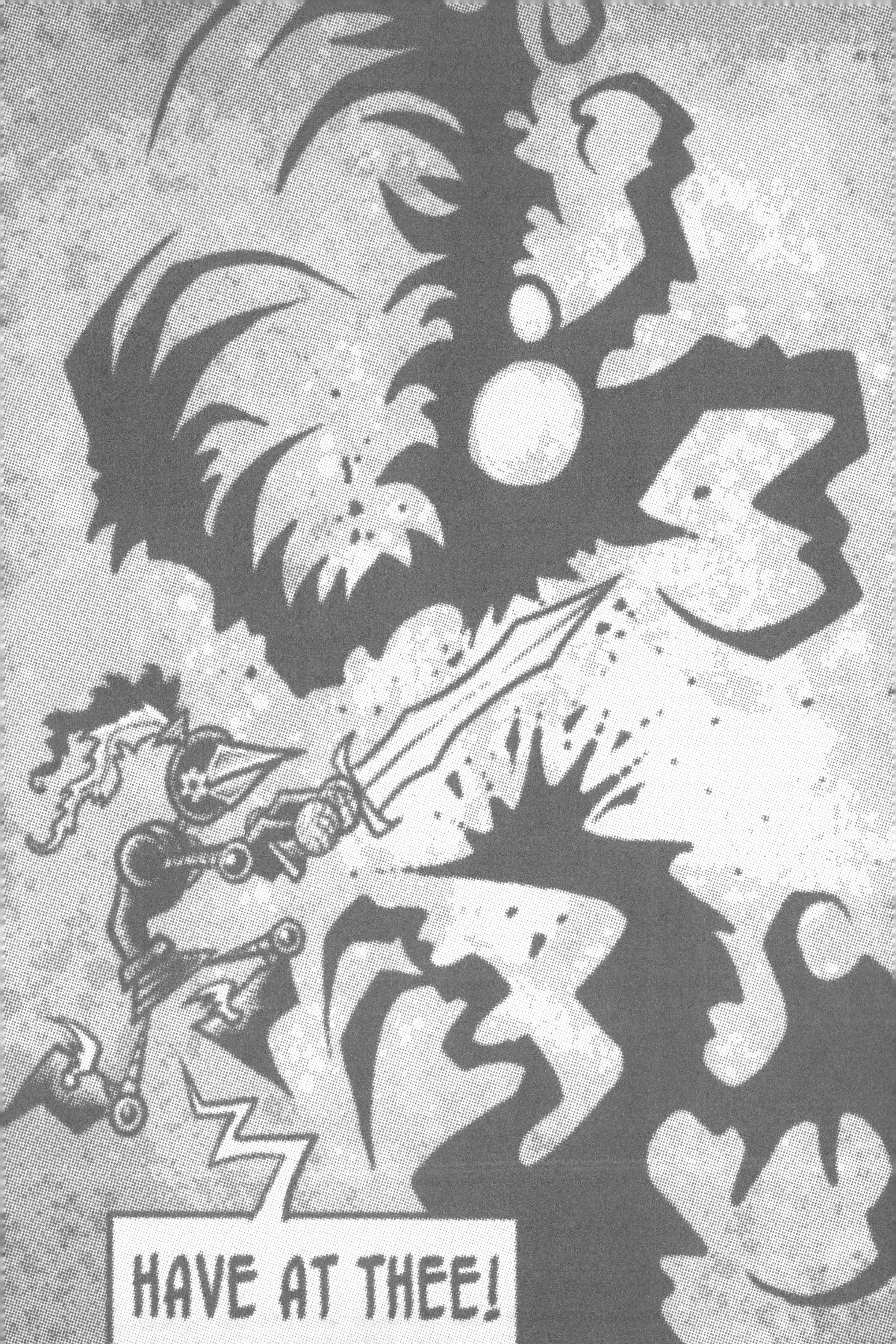
HAVE AT THEE!

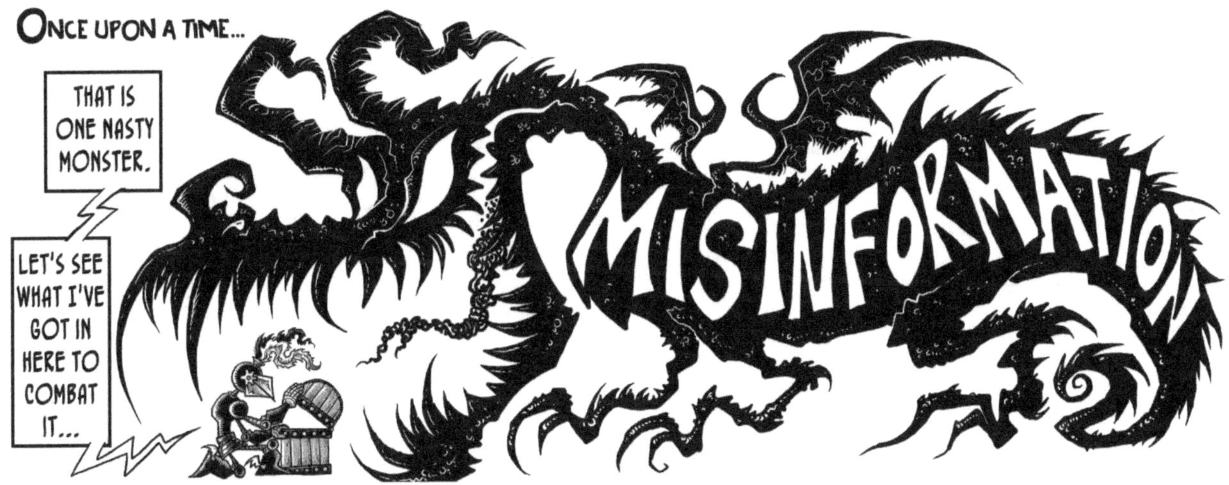

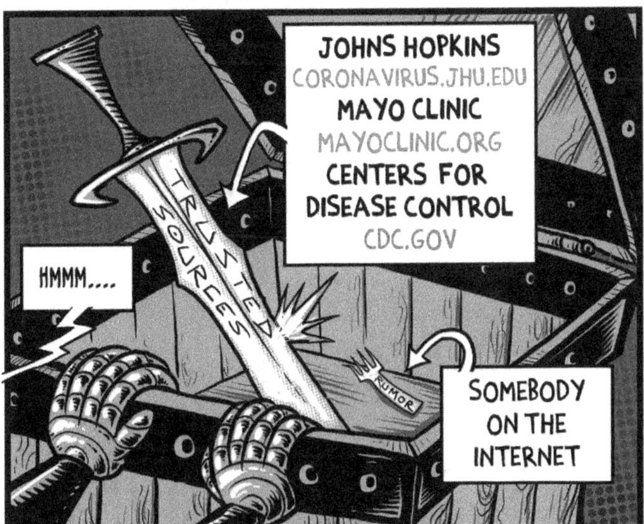

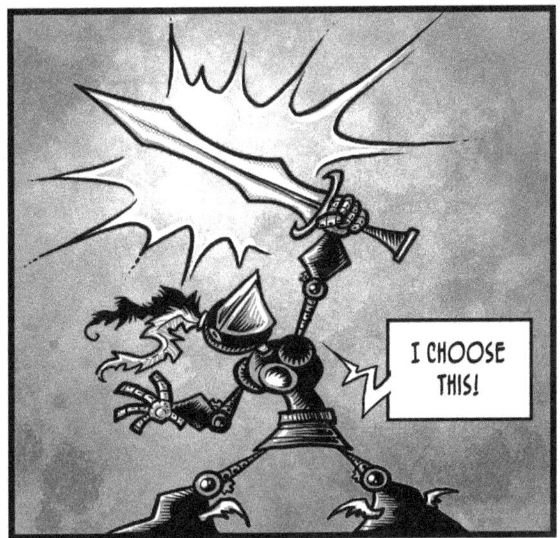

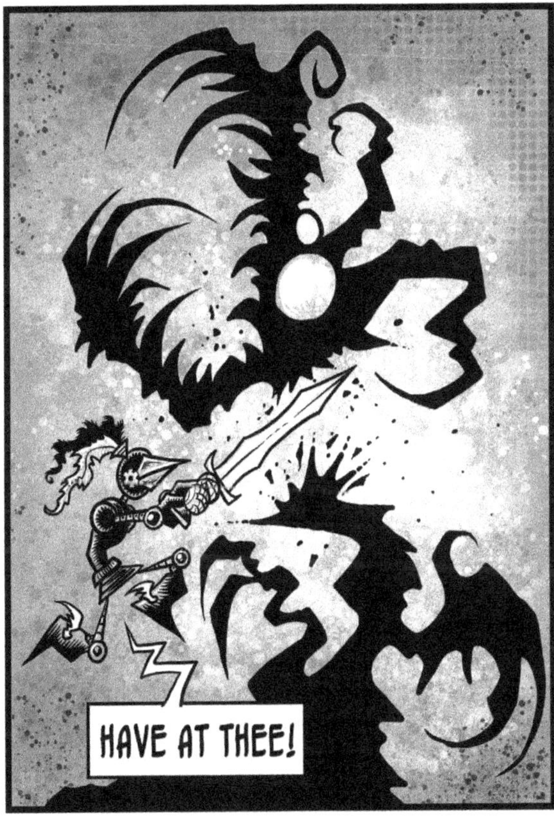

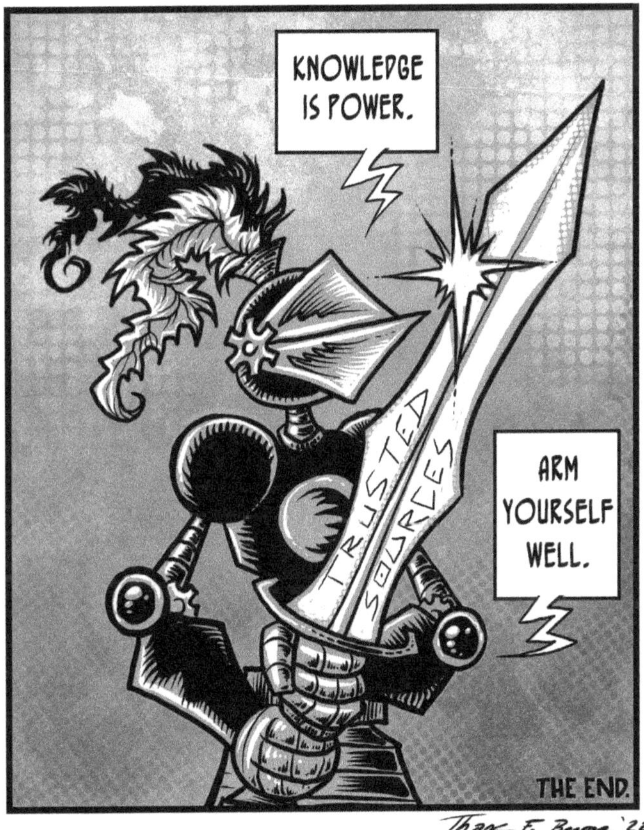

Art by Thane Benson.

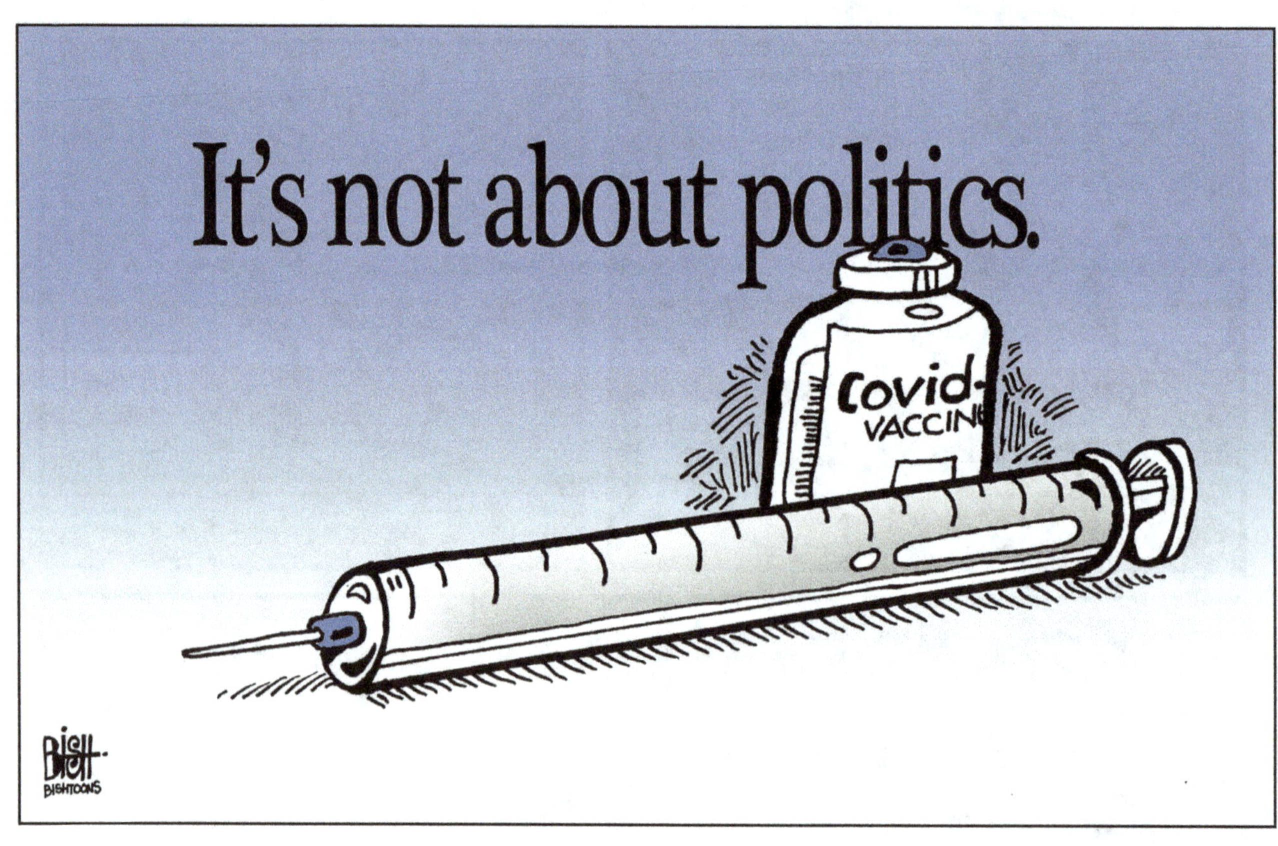

Art by Randy Bish.

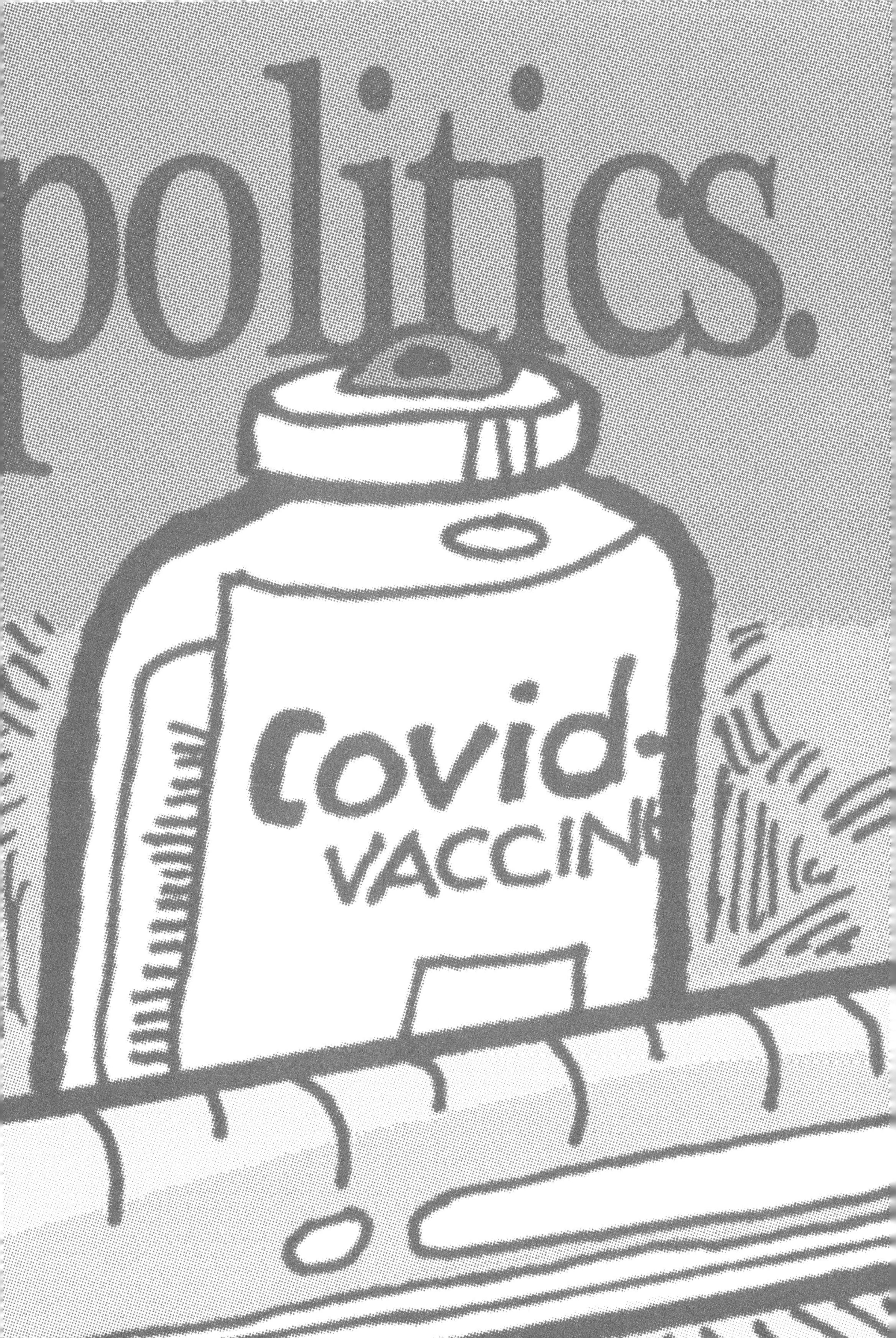
politics.
Covid-
VACCIN

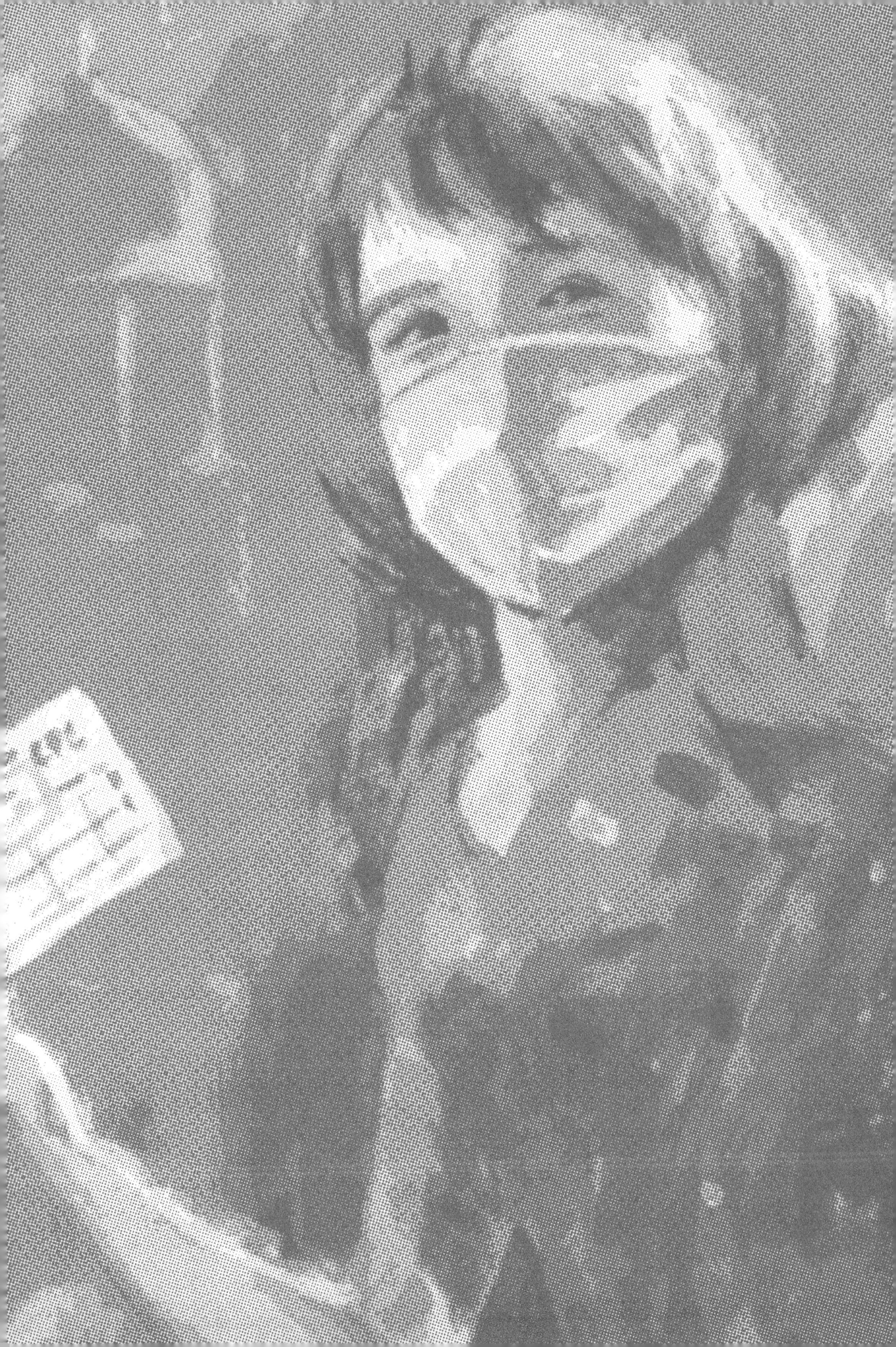

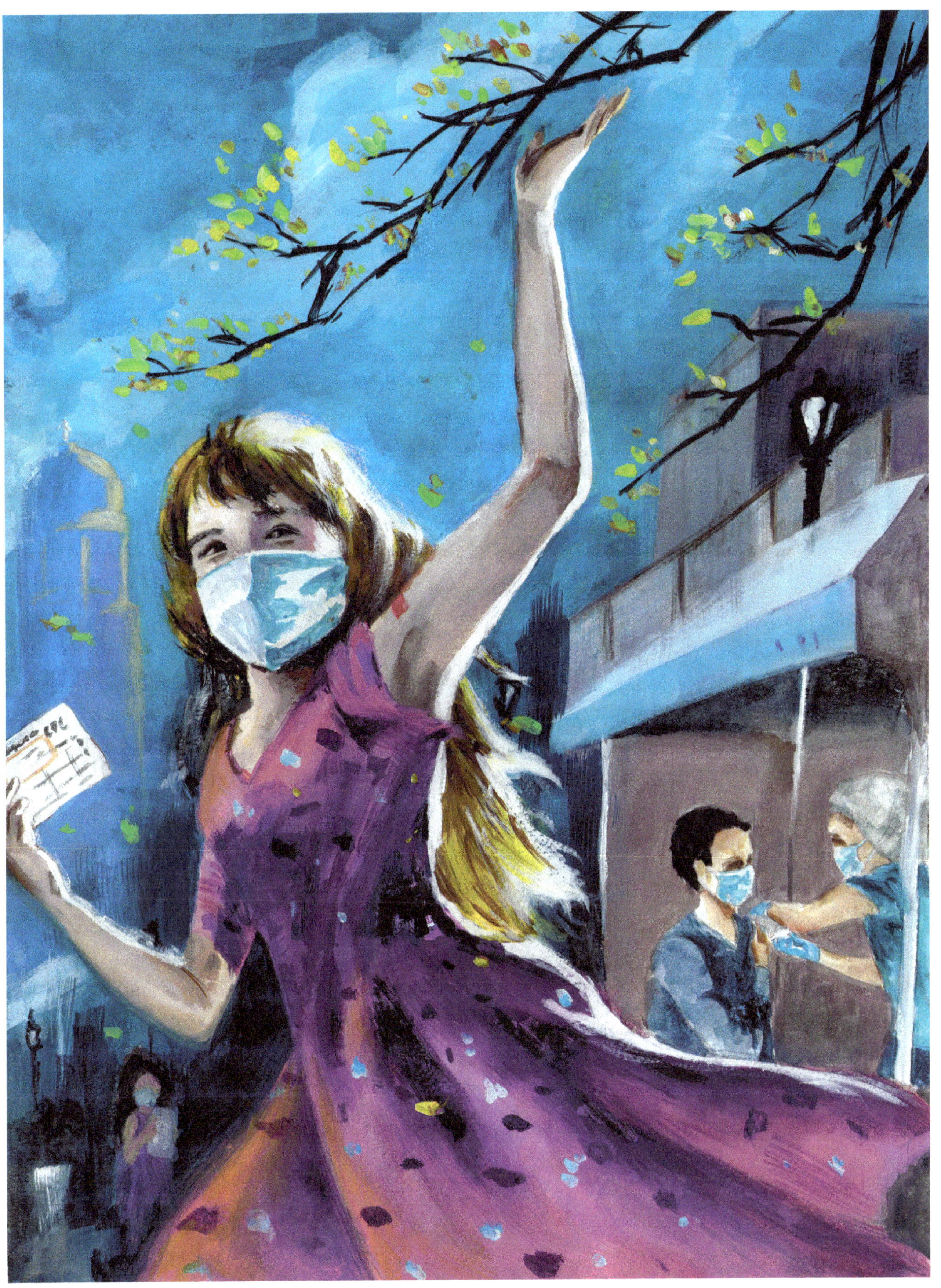

Art by Yihang Meng.

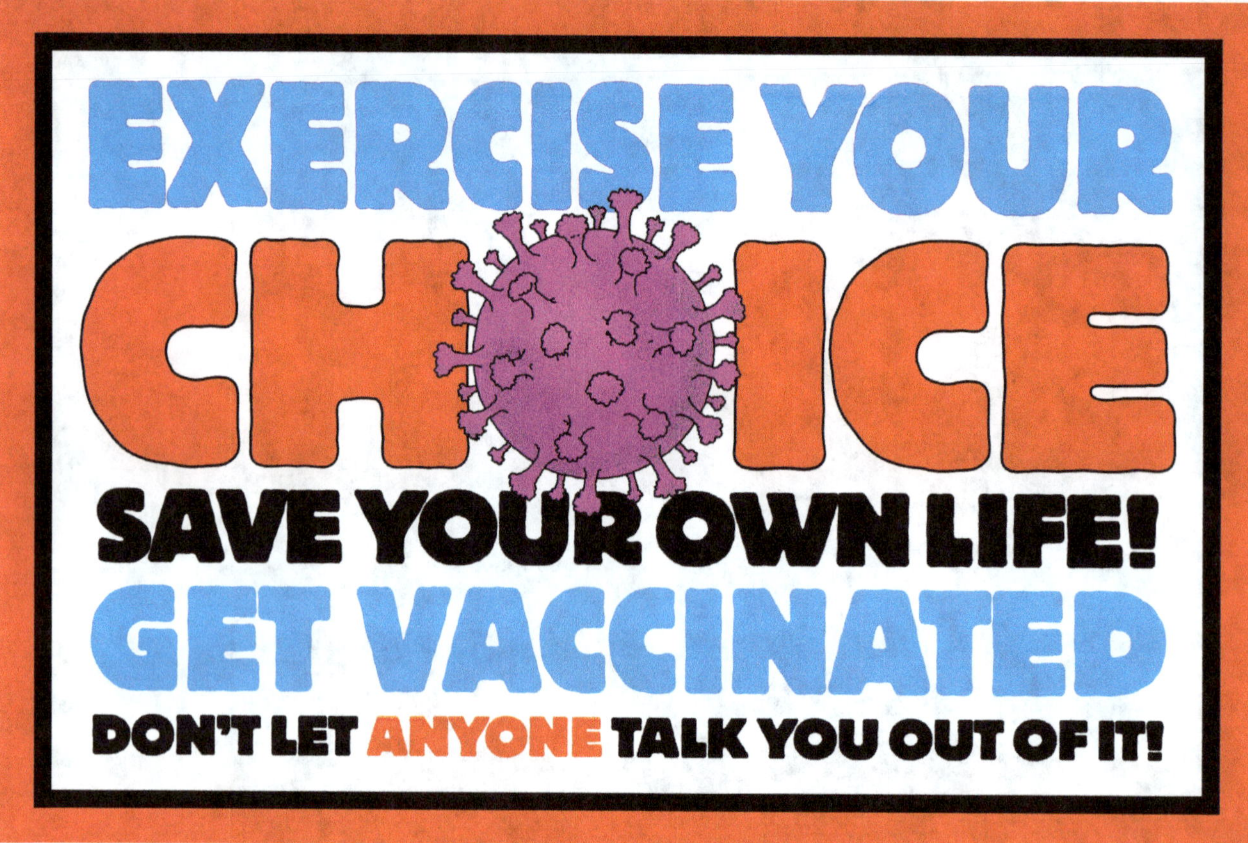

Art by William Wells.

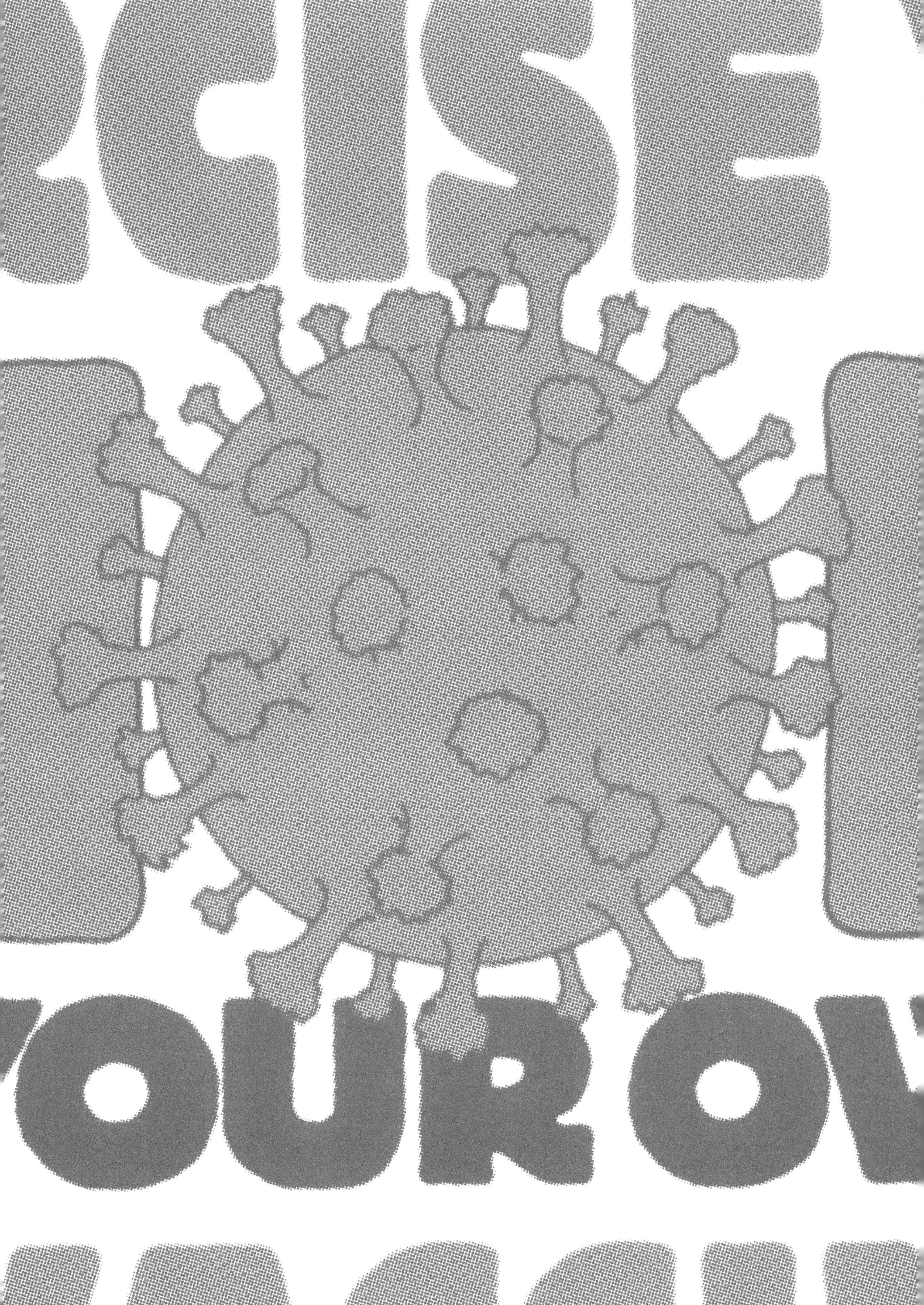
YOUR

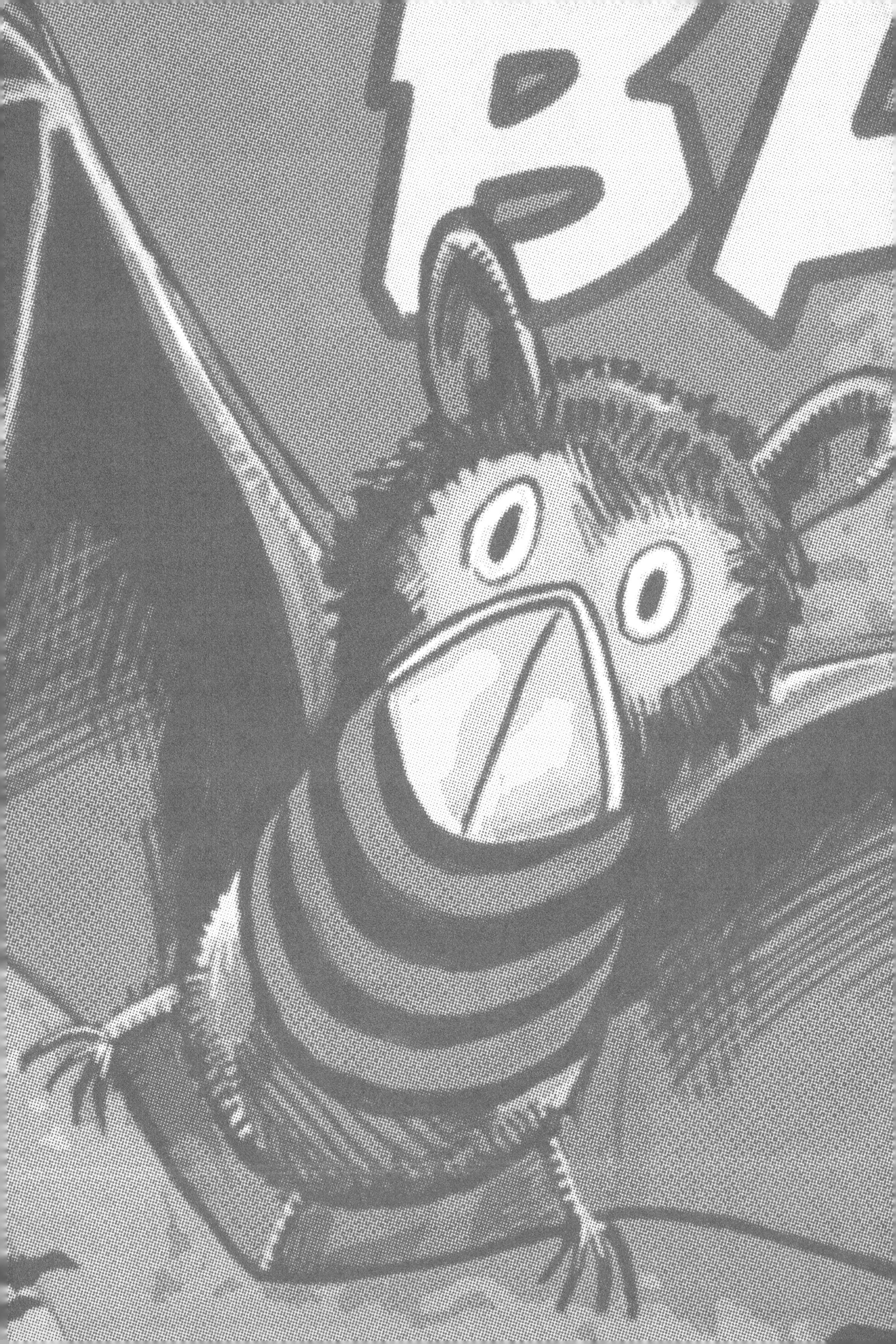

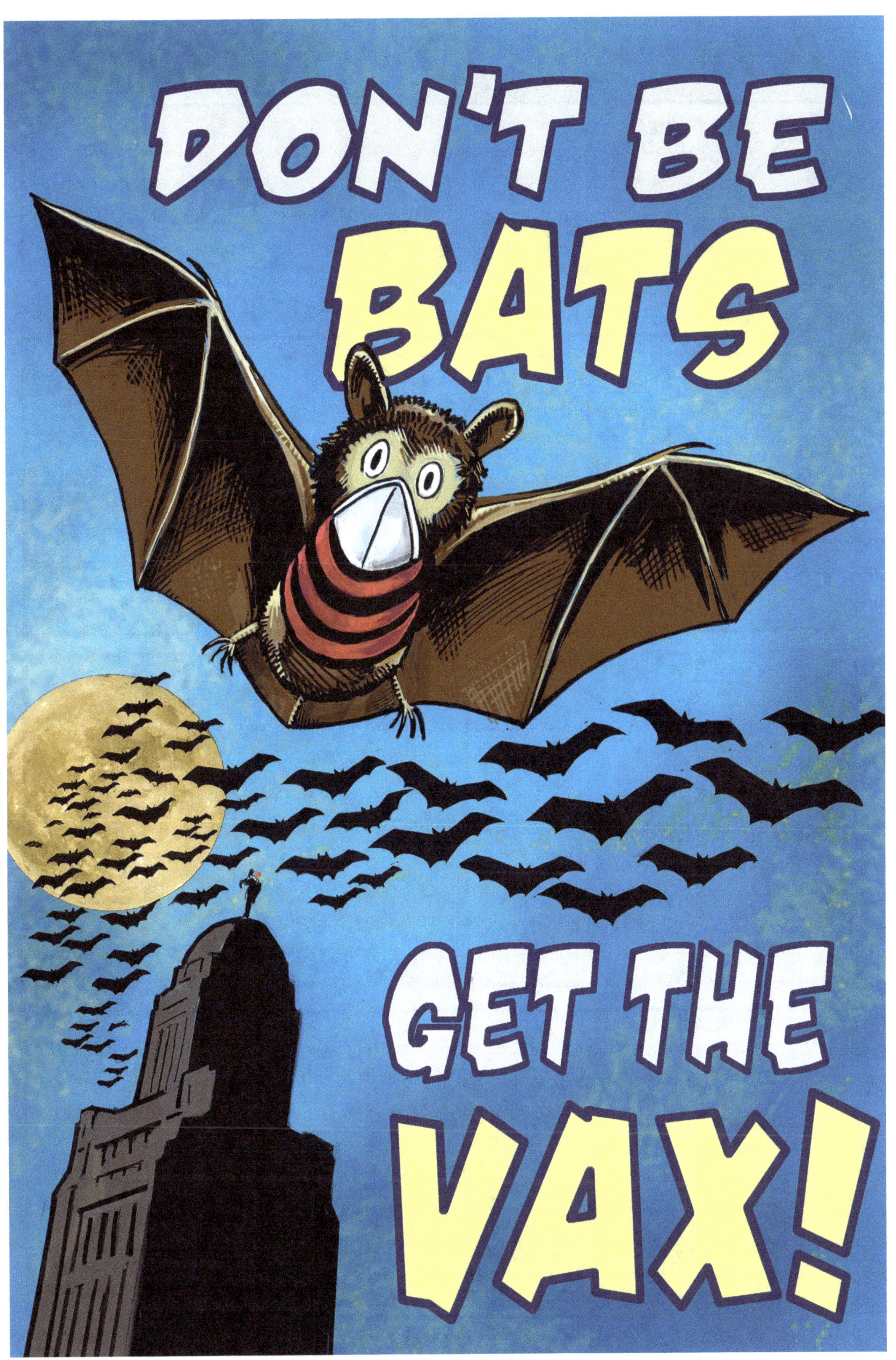

Art by Bob Hall.

AN OLD JOKE*

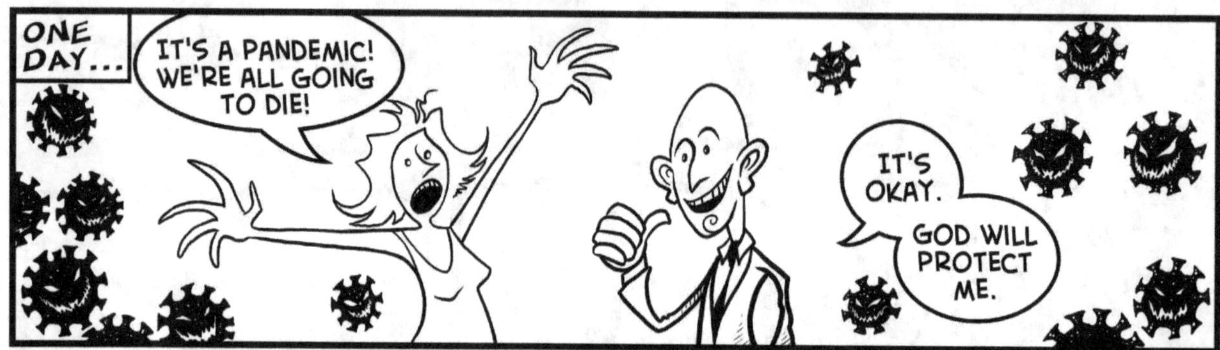

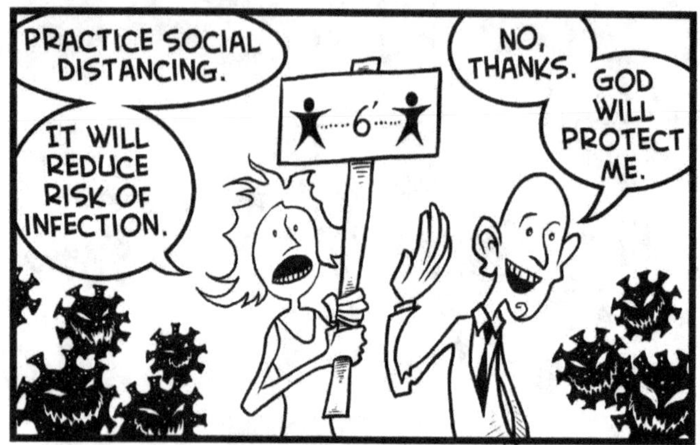

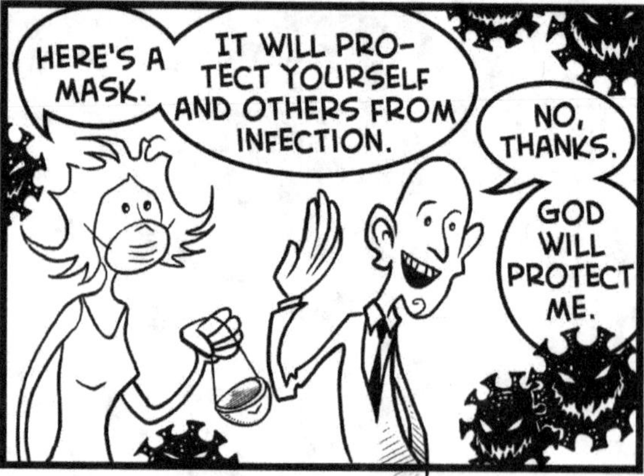

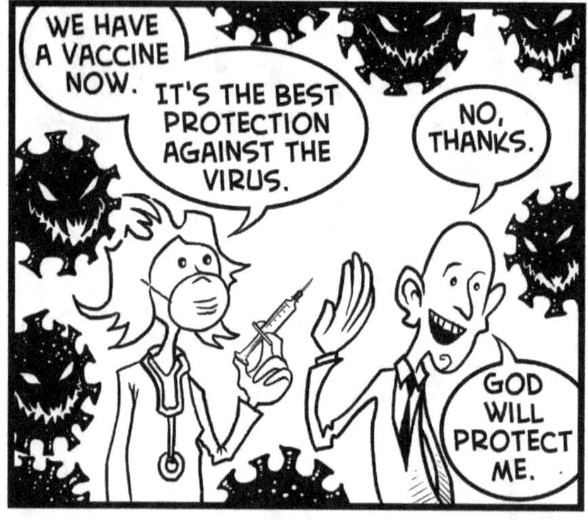

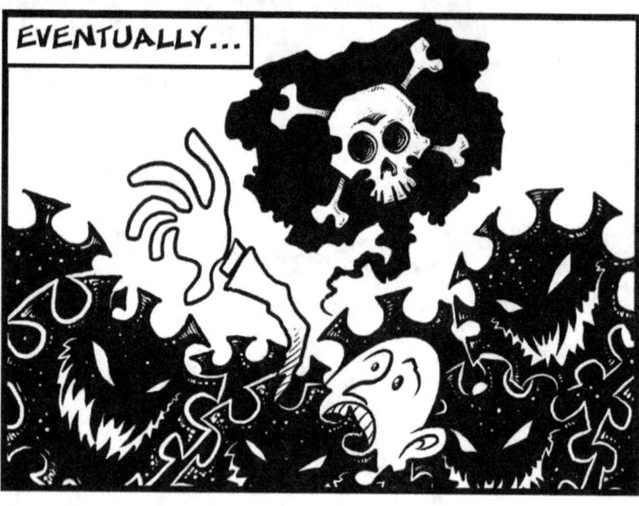

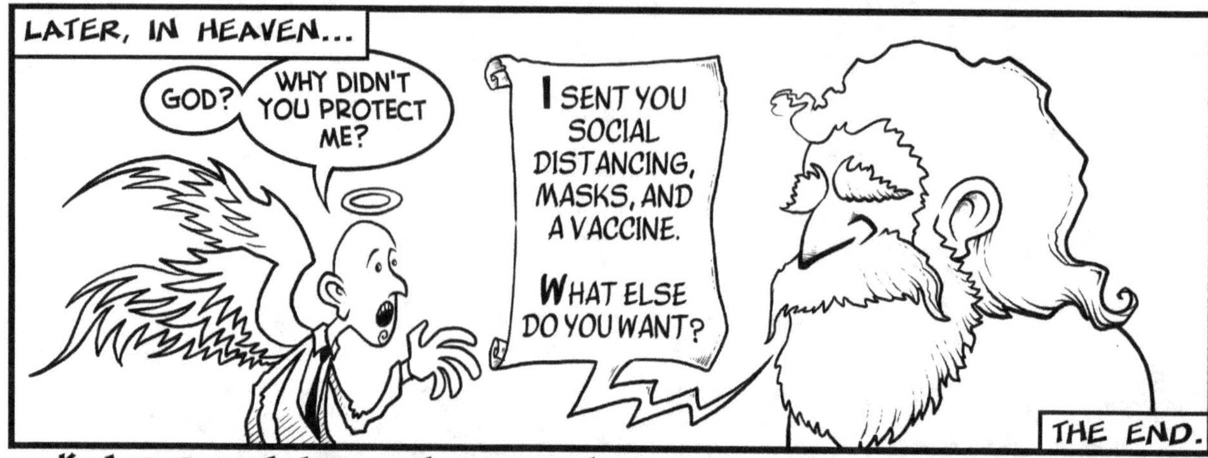

*UPDATED FOR MODERN TIMES

Art by Thane Benson.

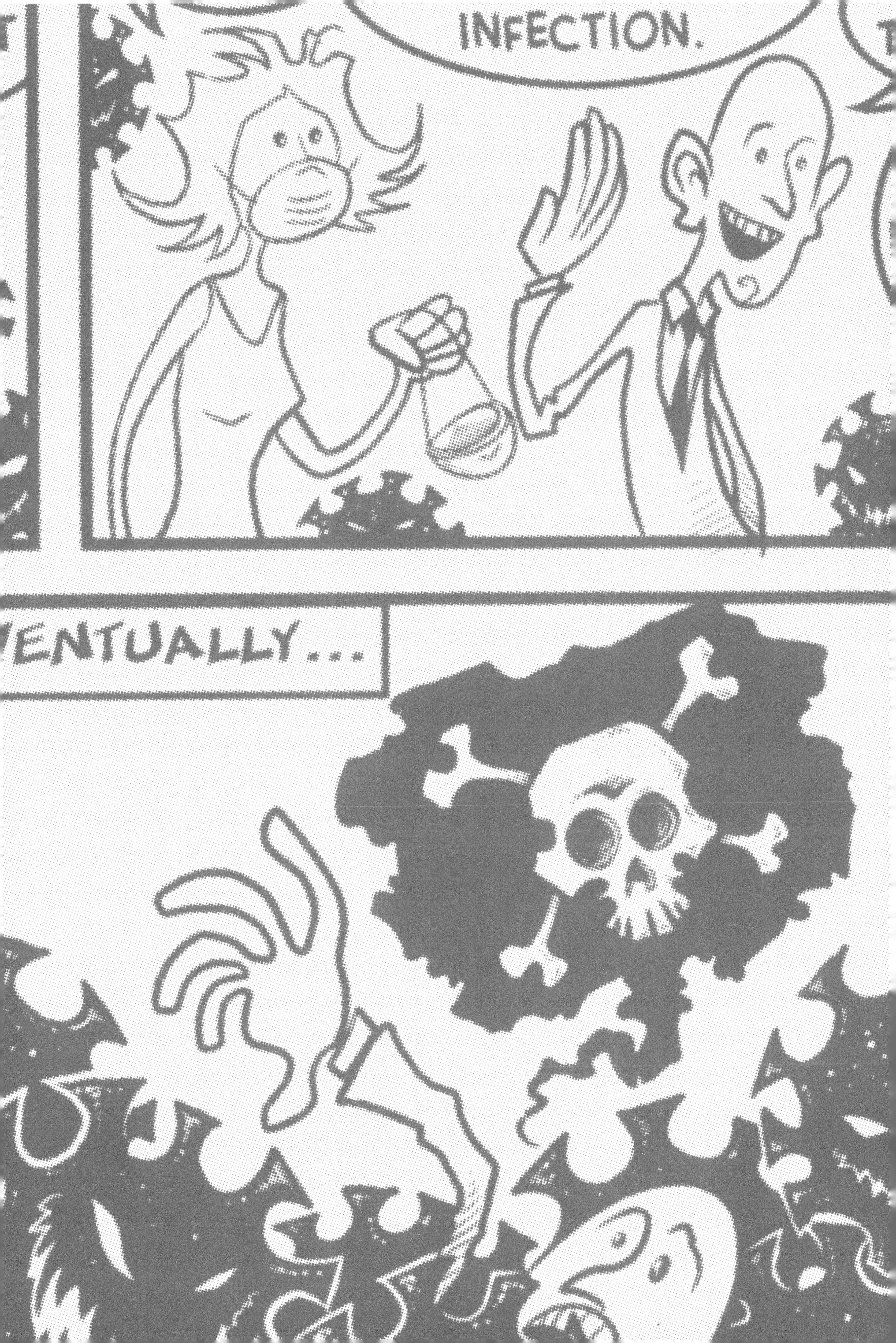

INFECTION.

ENTUALLY...

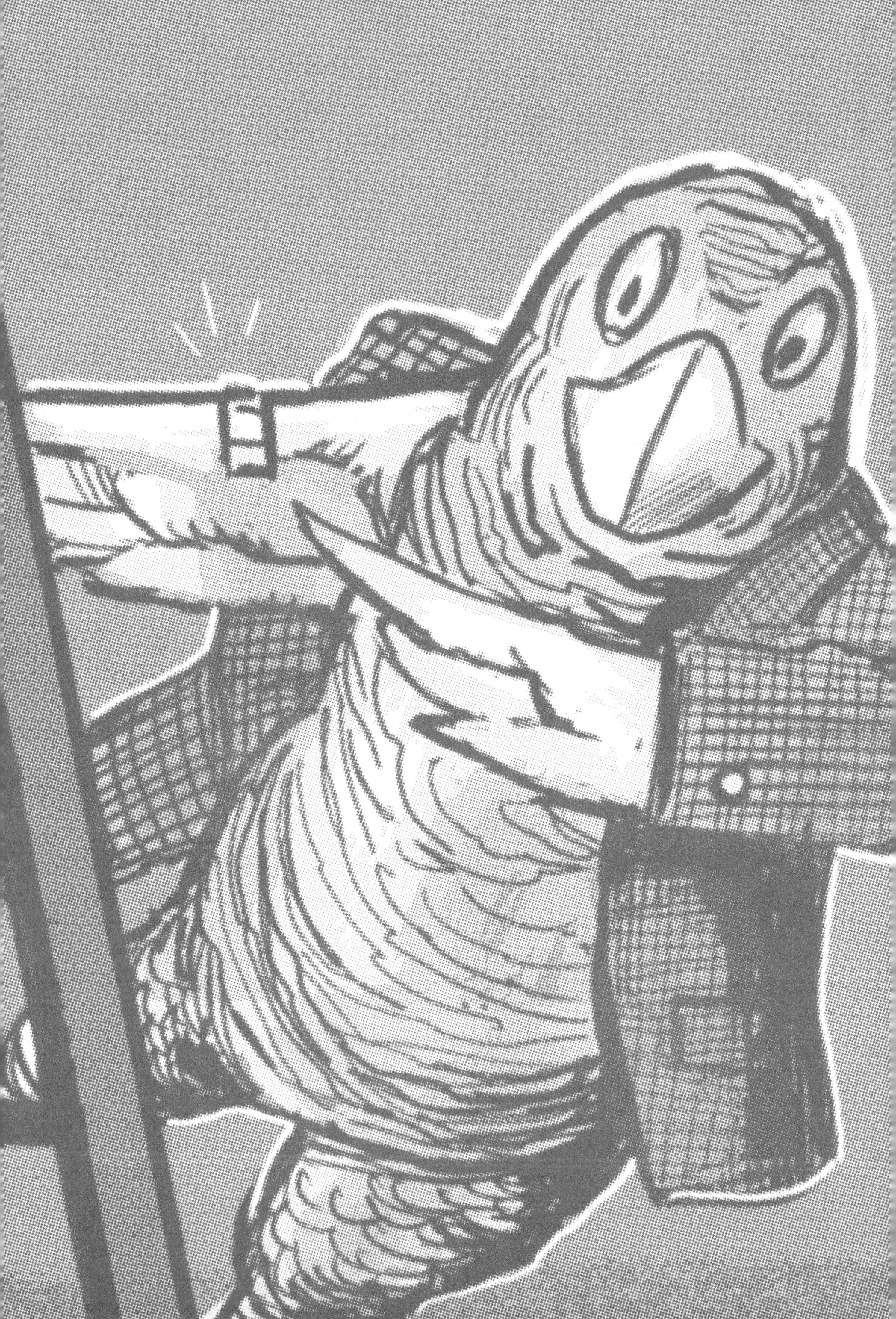

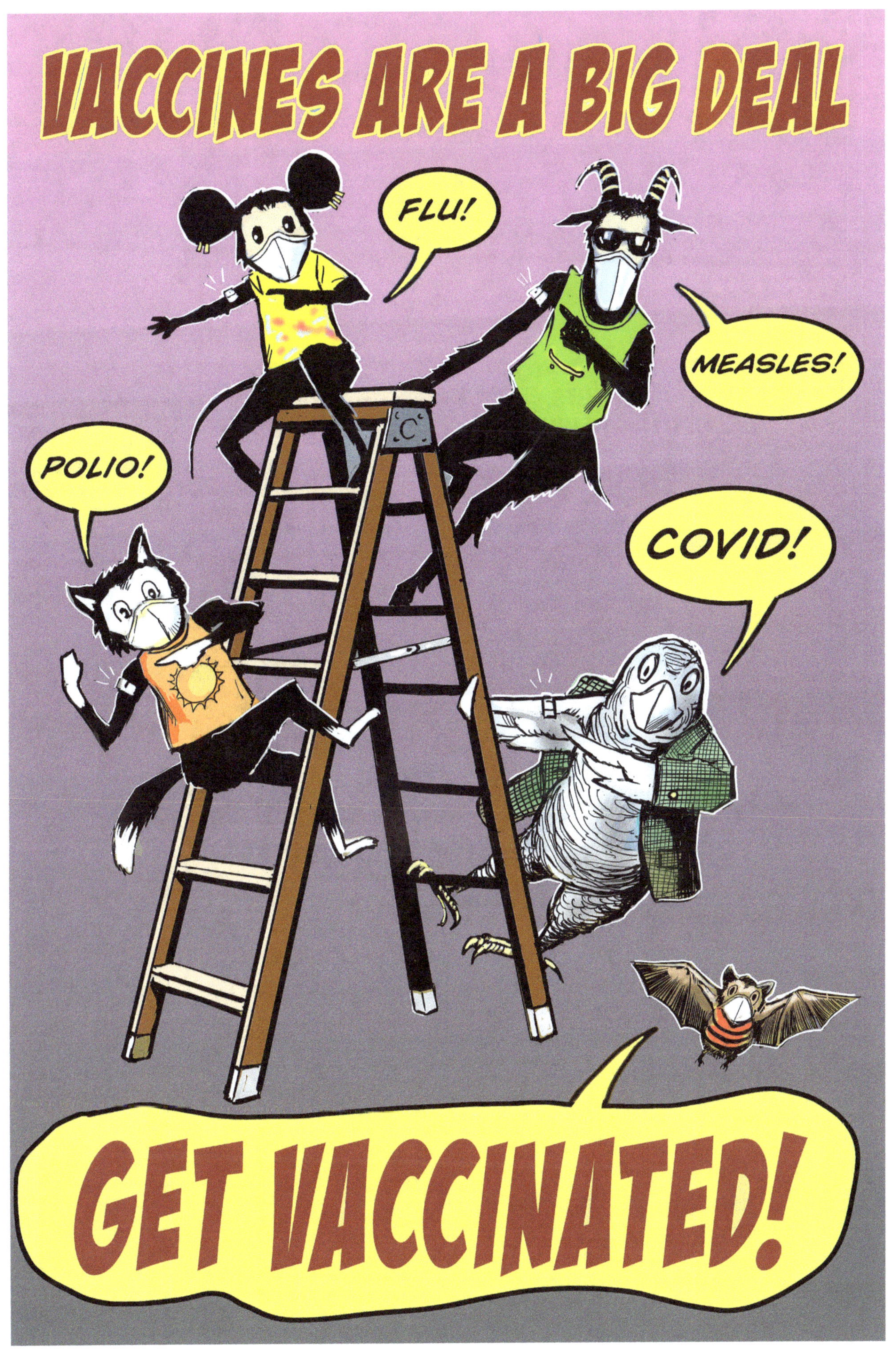

Art by Bob Hall.

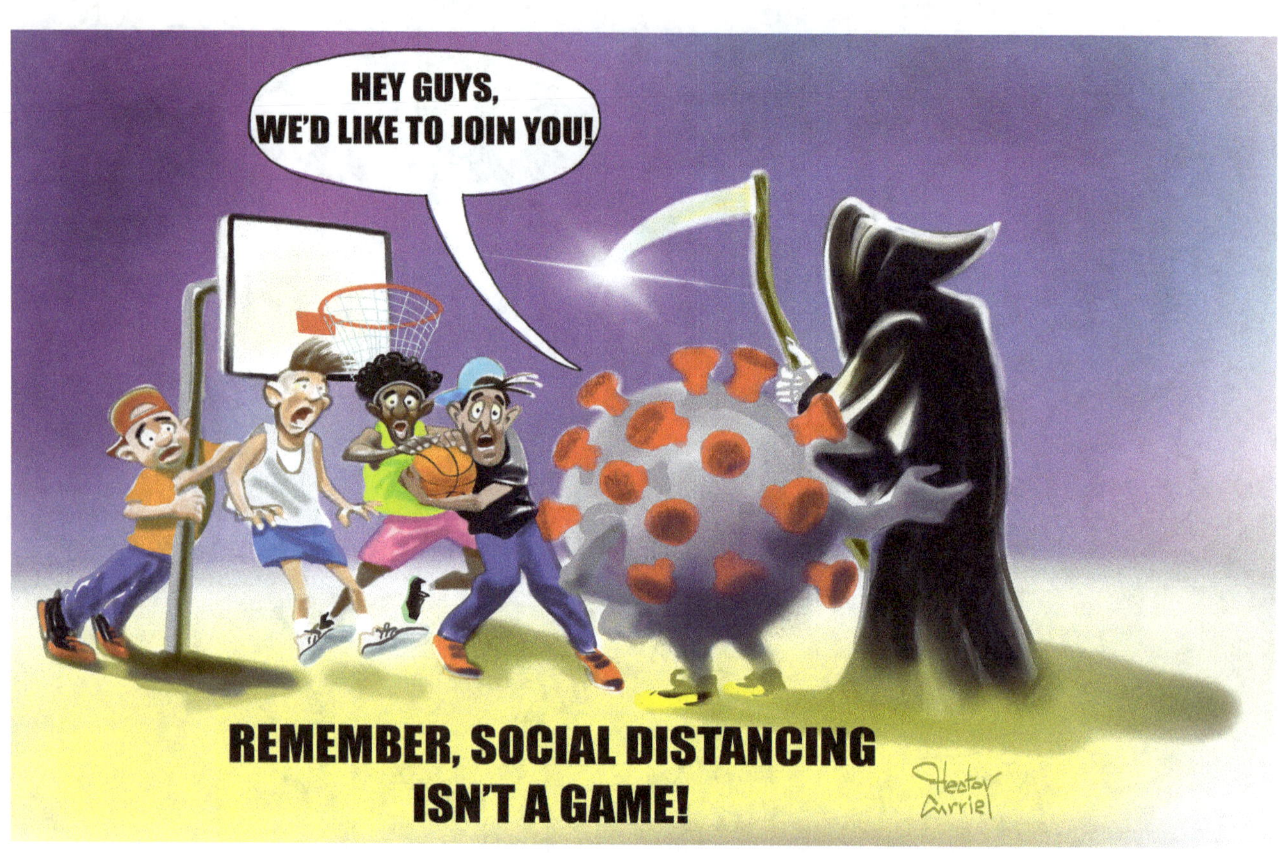

Art by Hector Curriel.

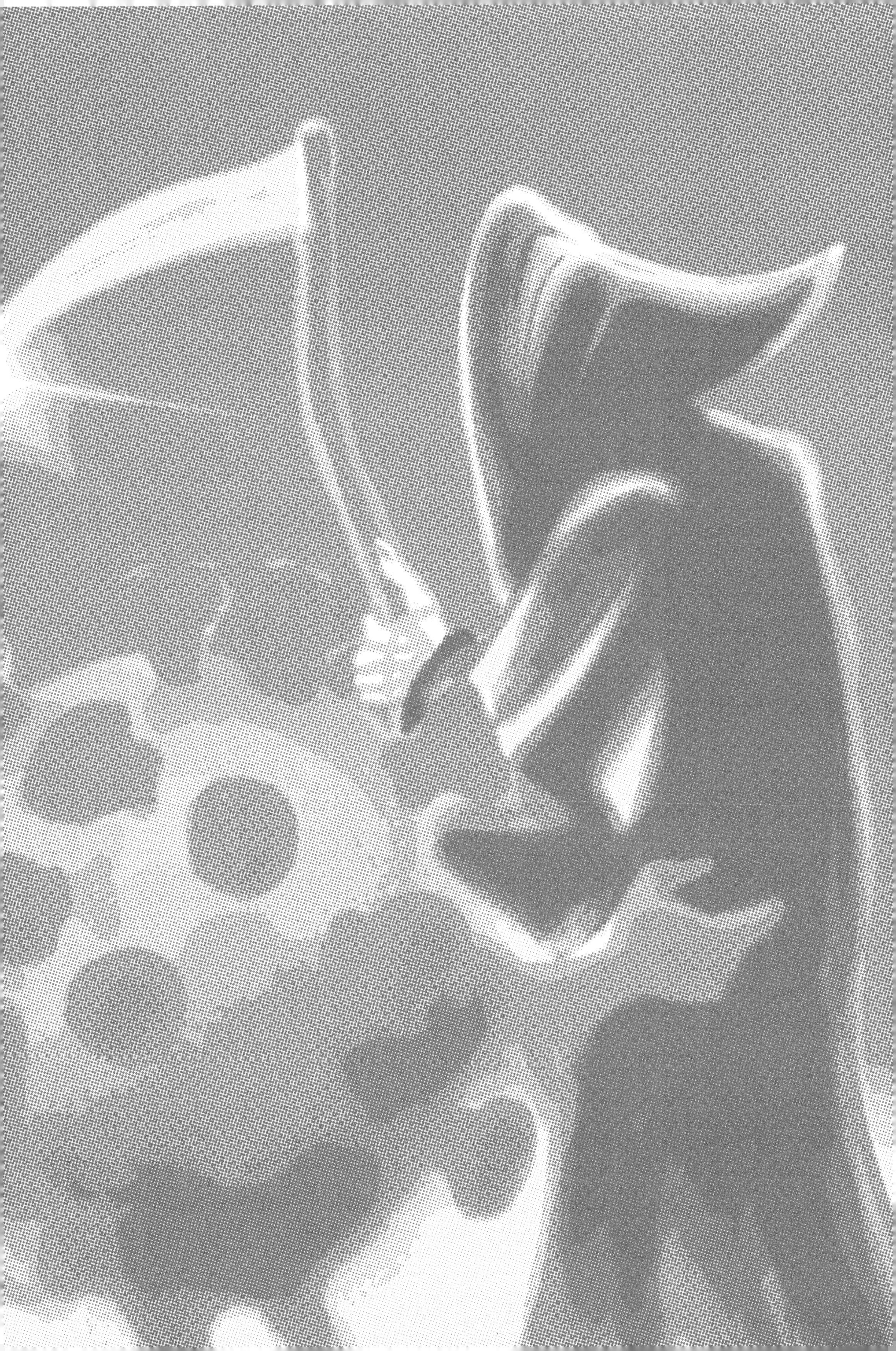

Prevent Vaccine Hesitancy

Learn to tell Vaccine FACT from MYTH

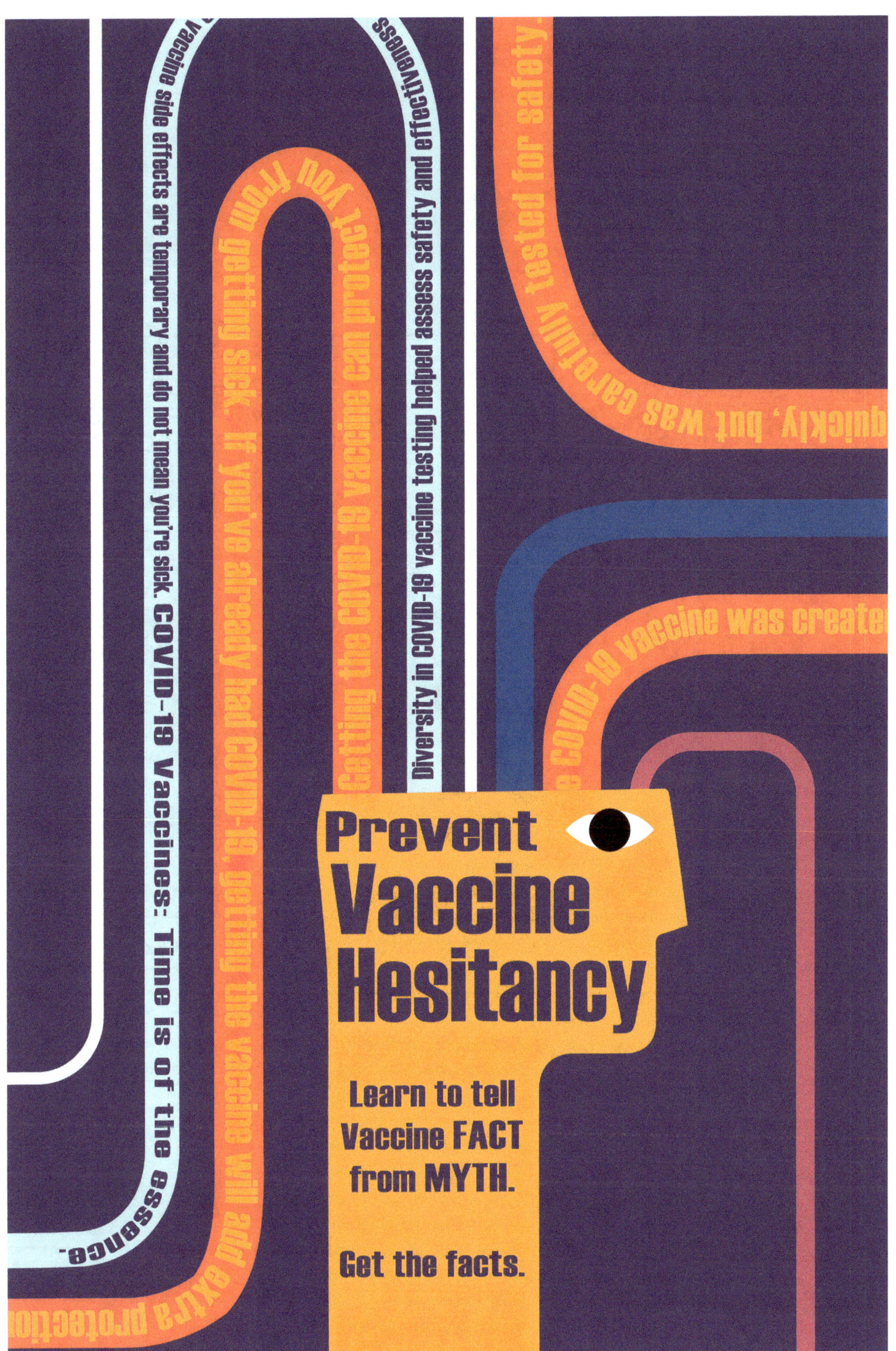

Art by Rachel Claire Balter.

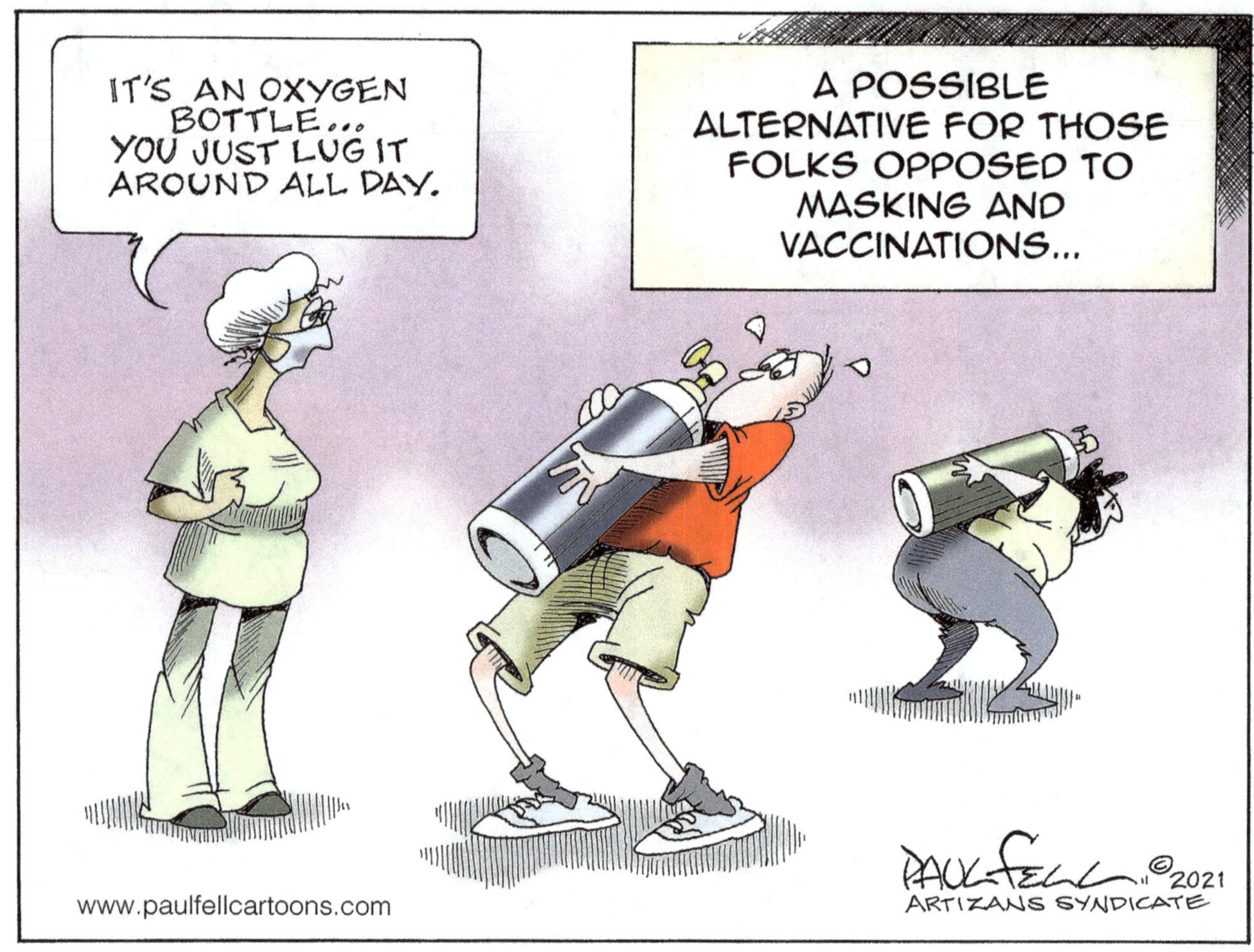

Art by Paul Fell.

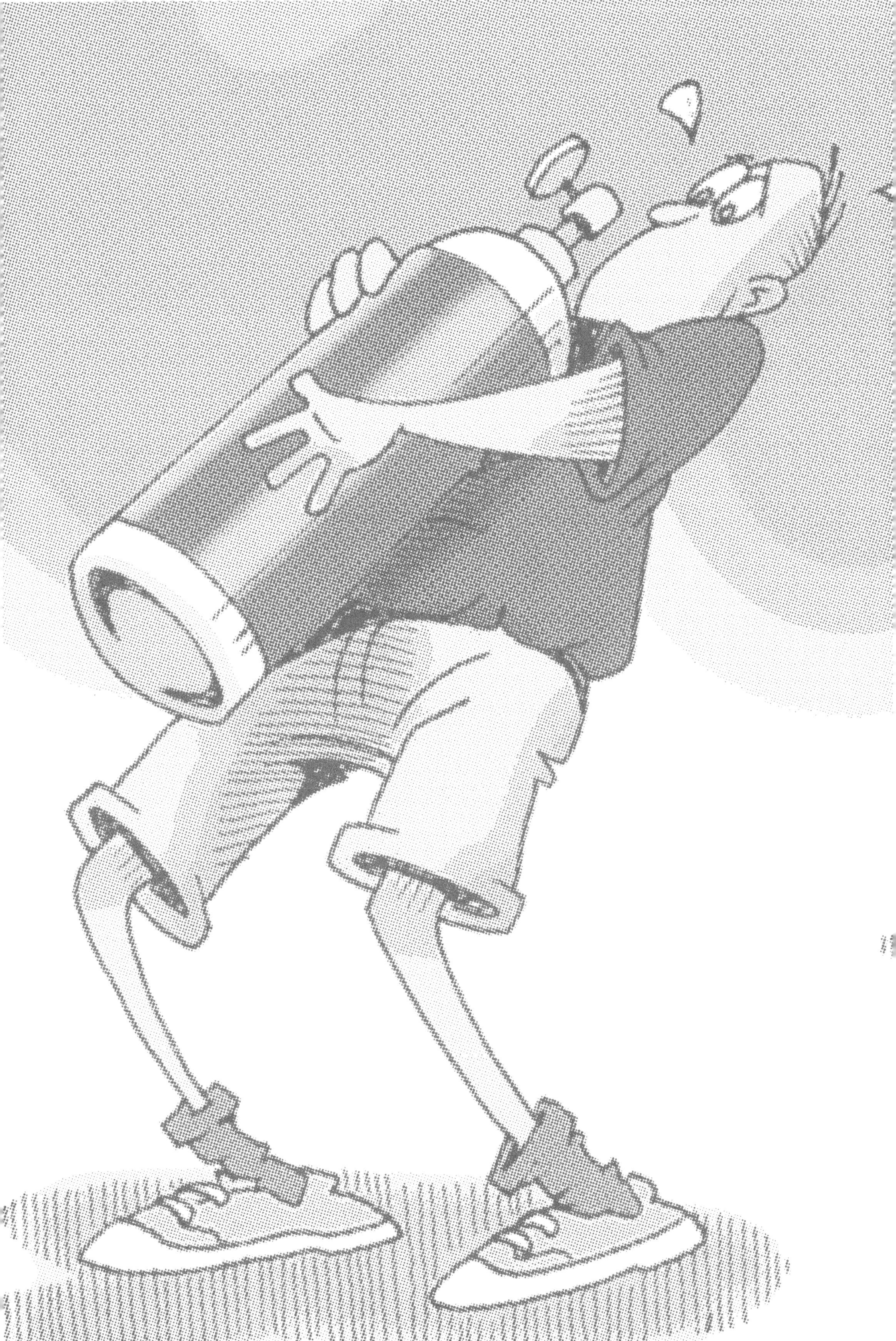

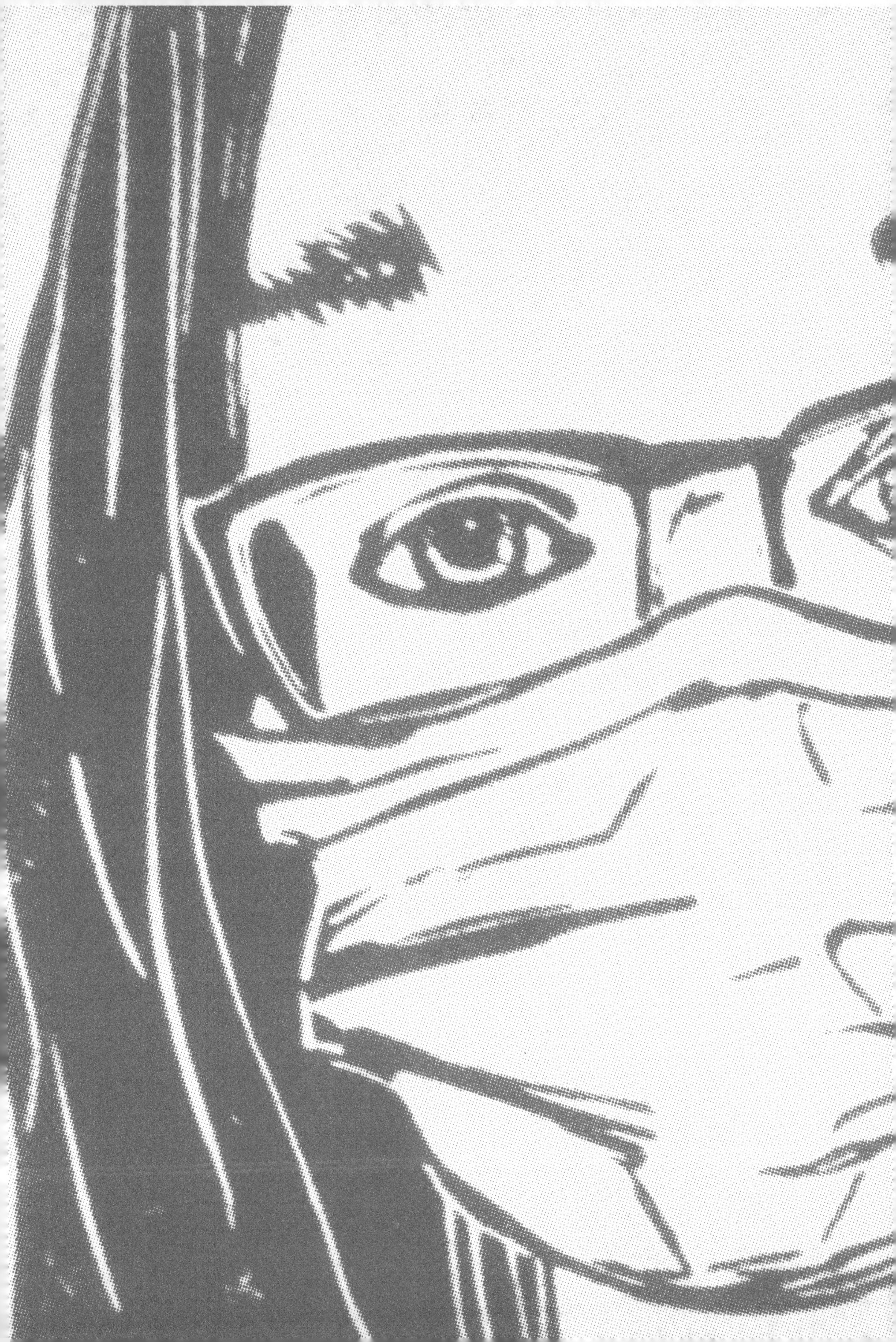

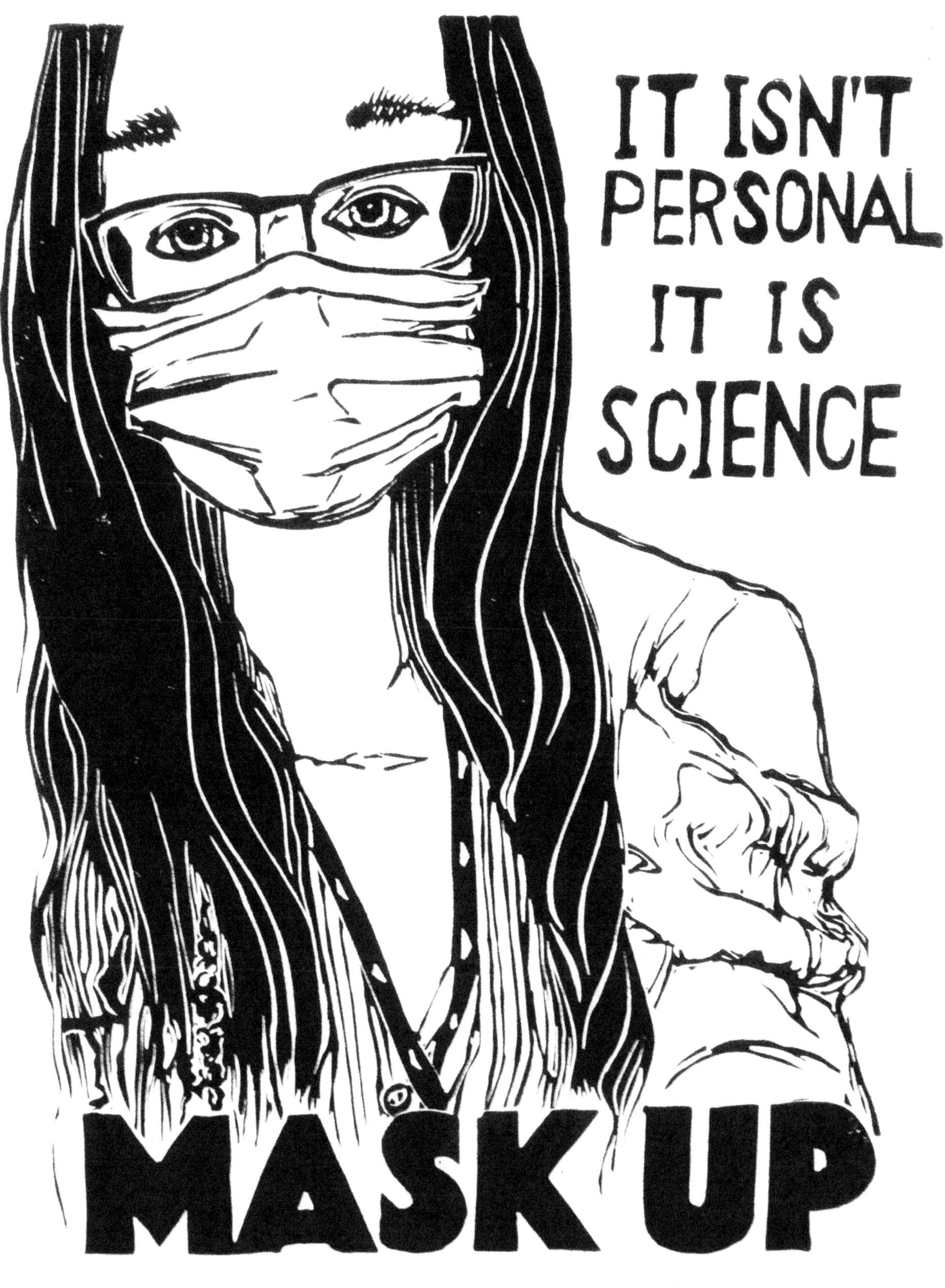

GET YOUR
COVID VACCINATIONS

Art by Ben Darling.

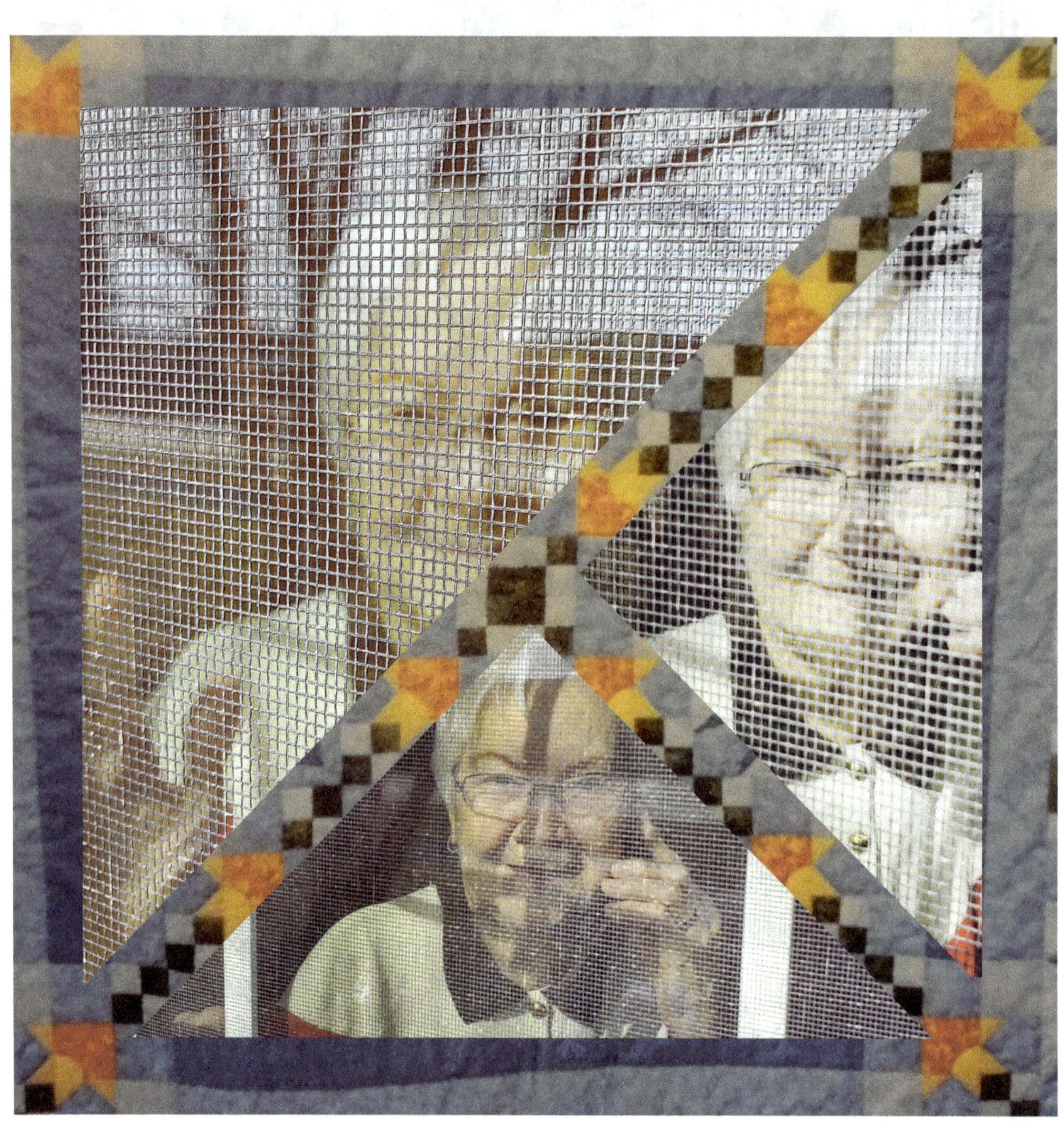

Art by Abbey Krienke.

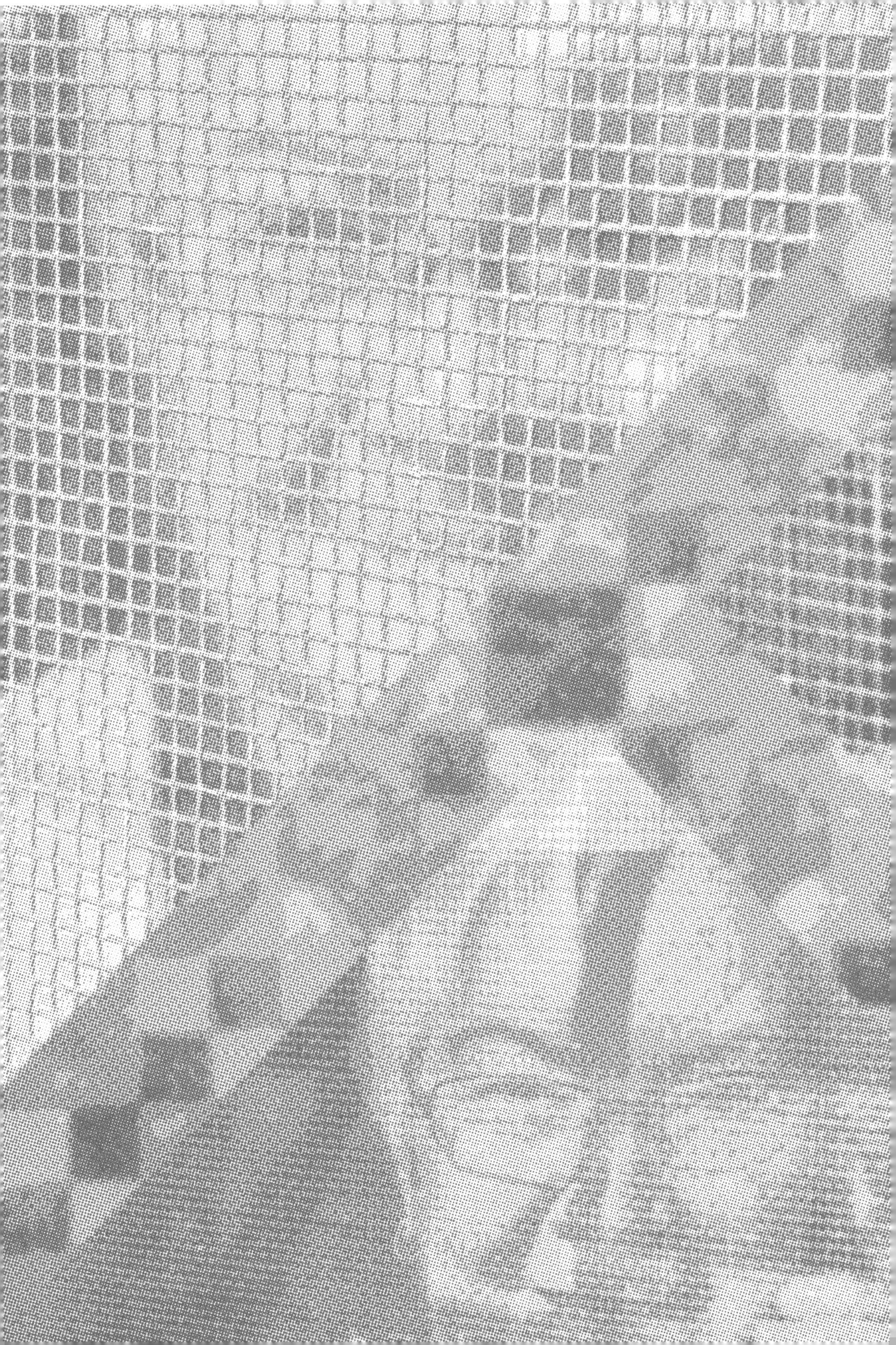

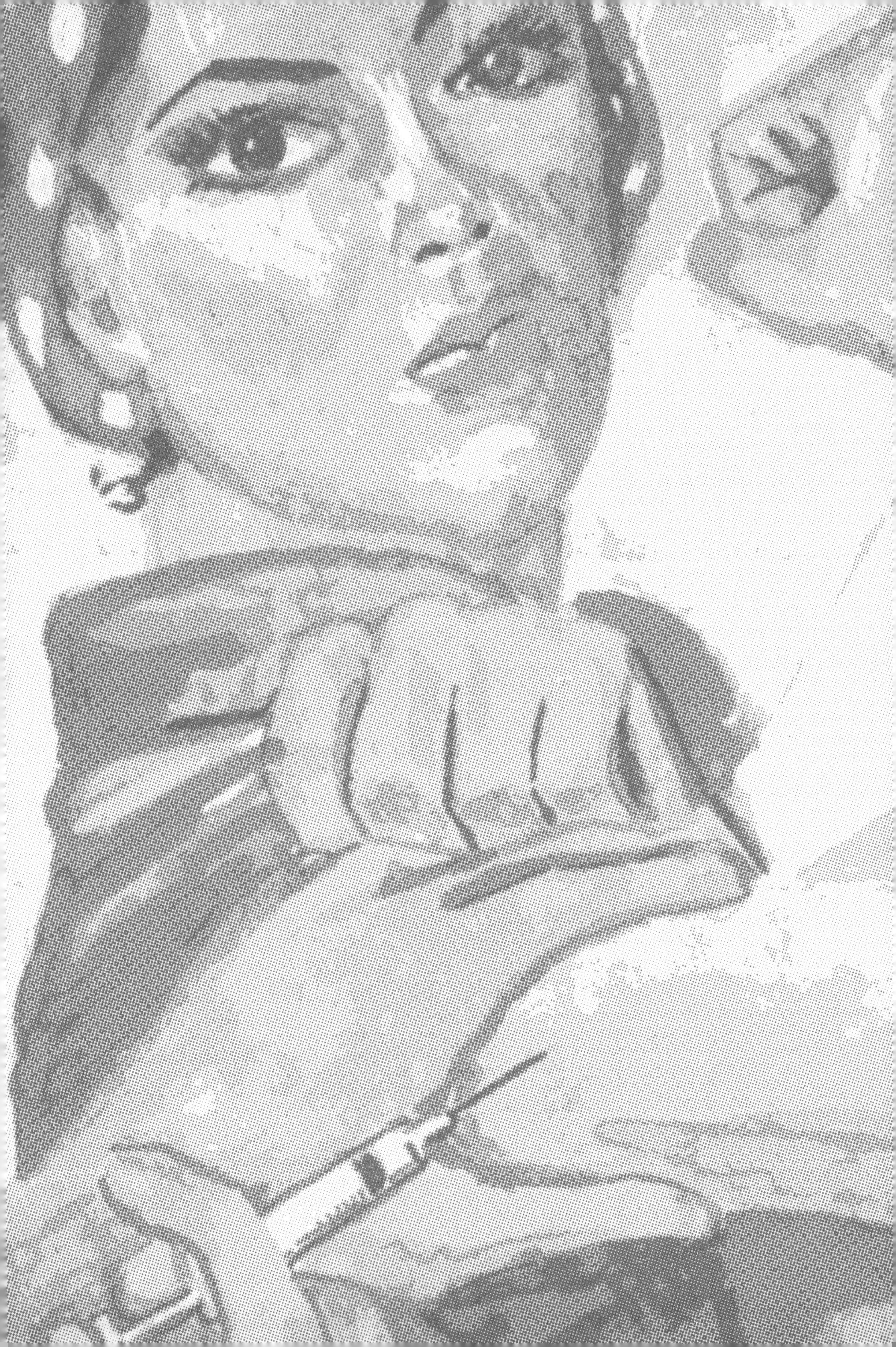

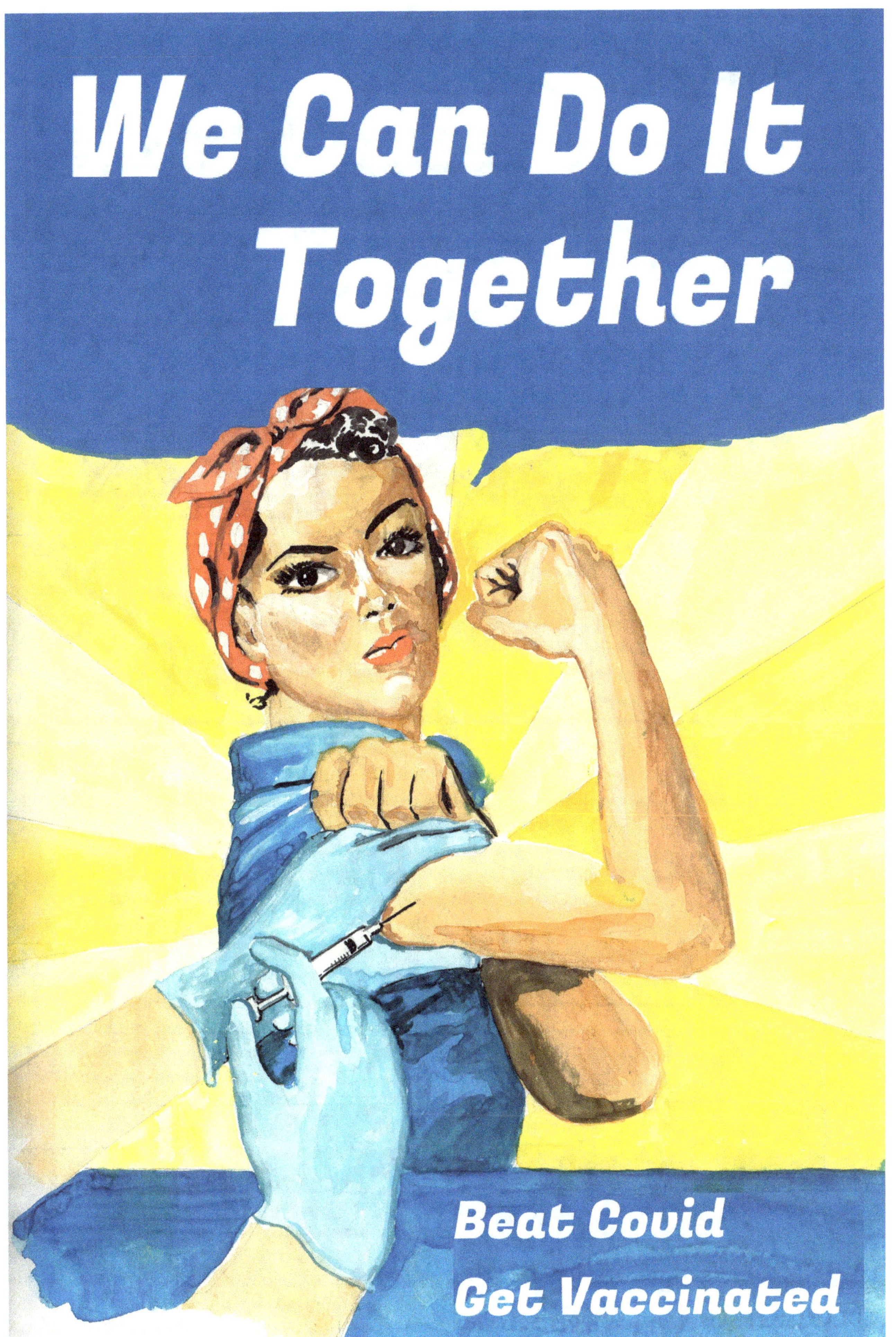

Art by David L Felley.

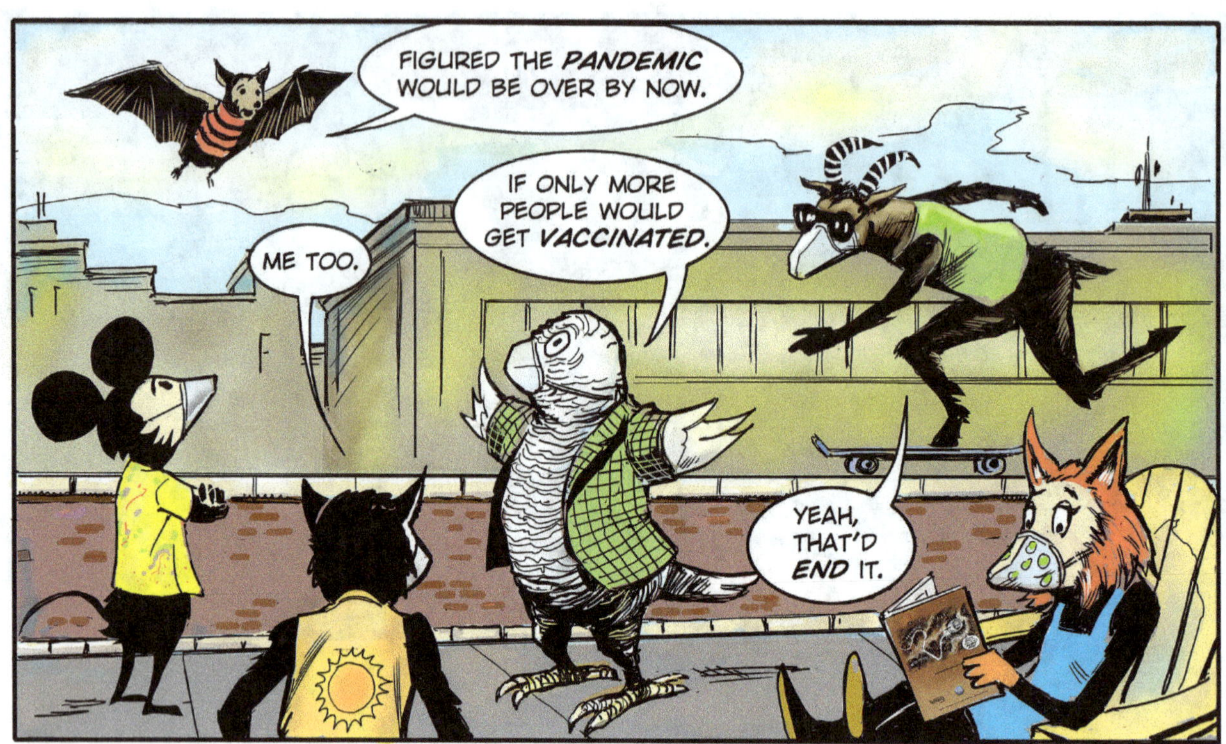

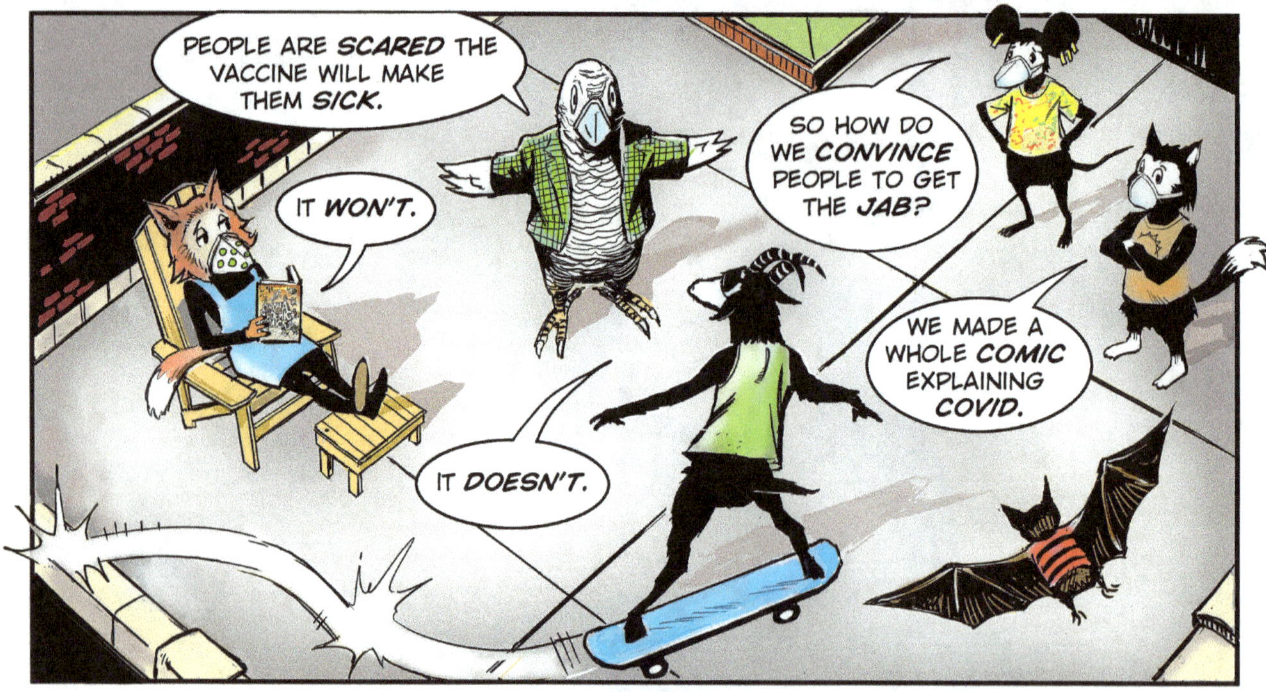

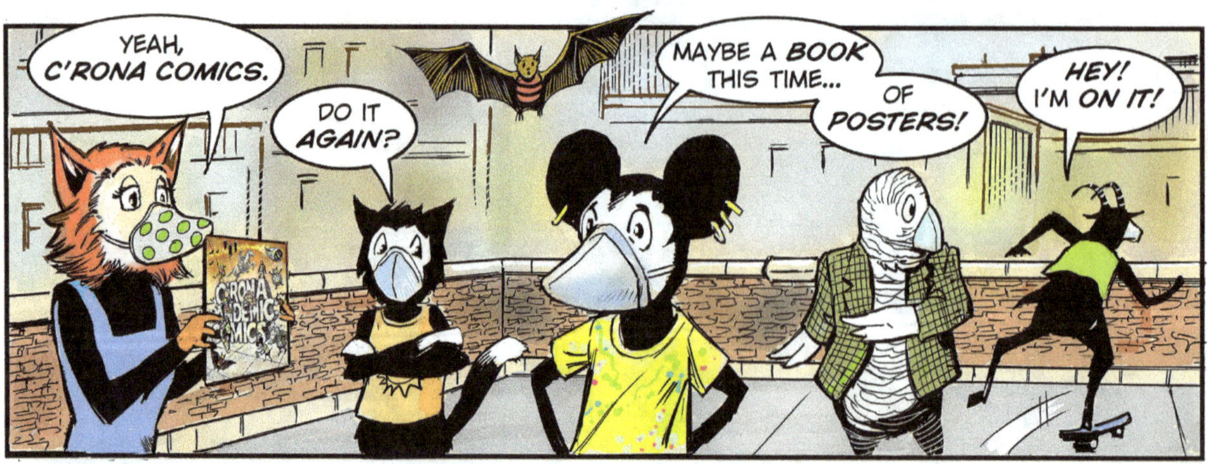

Art by Bob Hall.

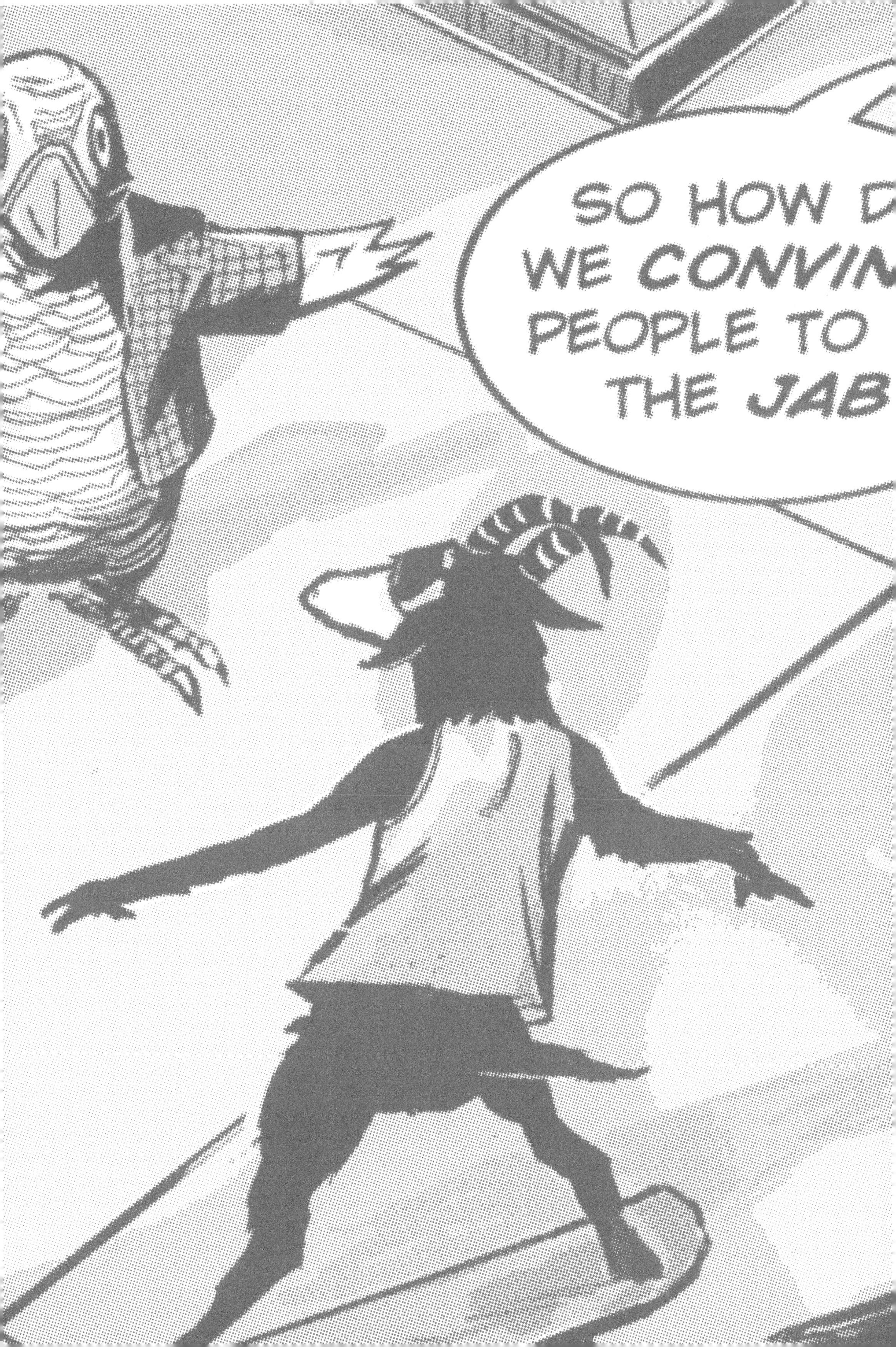
SO HOW D WE *CONVIN* PEOPLE TO THE *JAB*

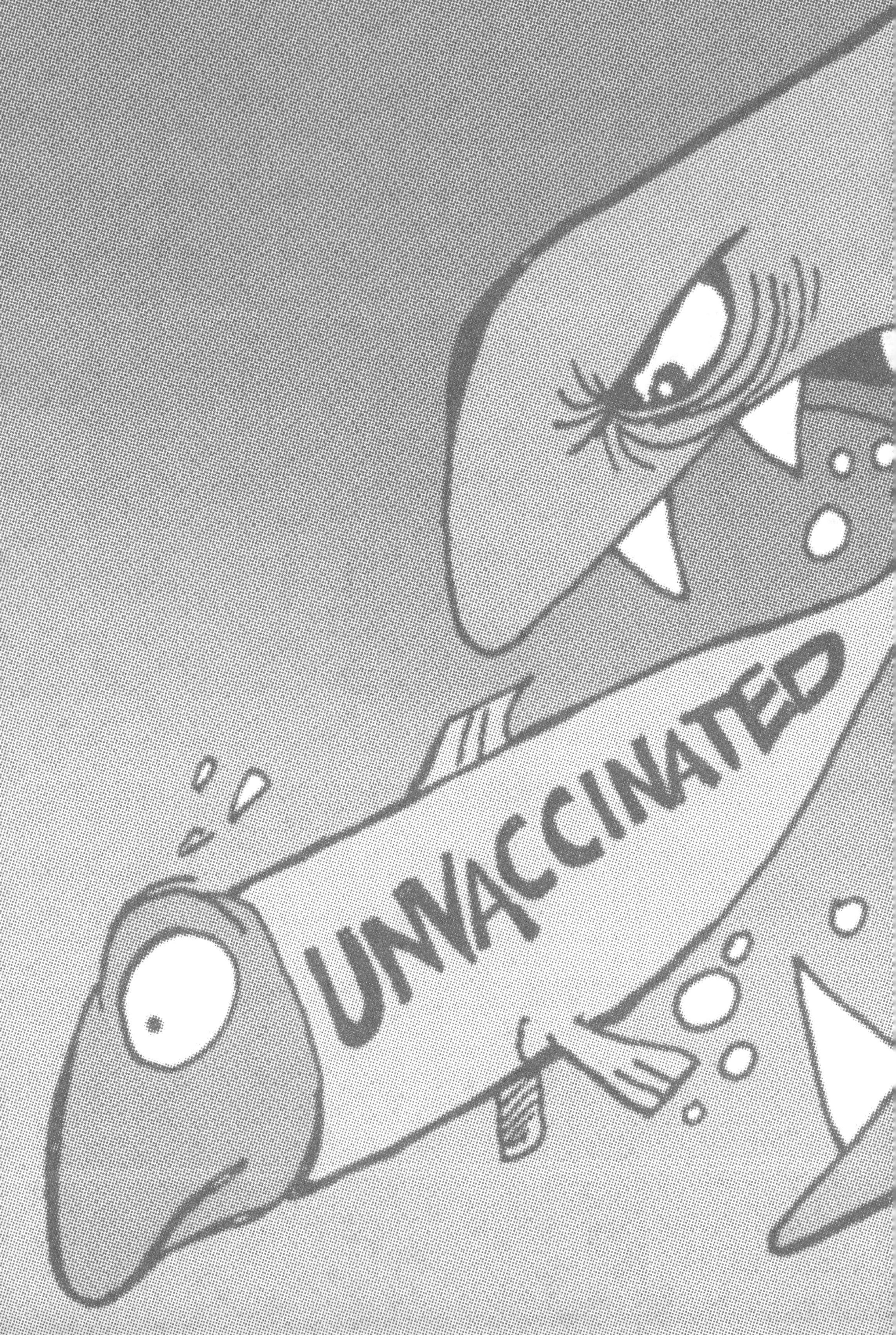
UNVACCINATED

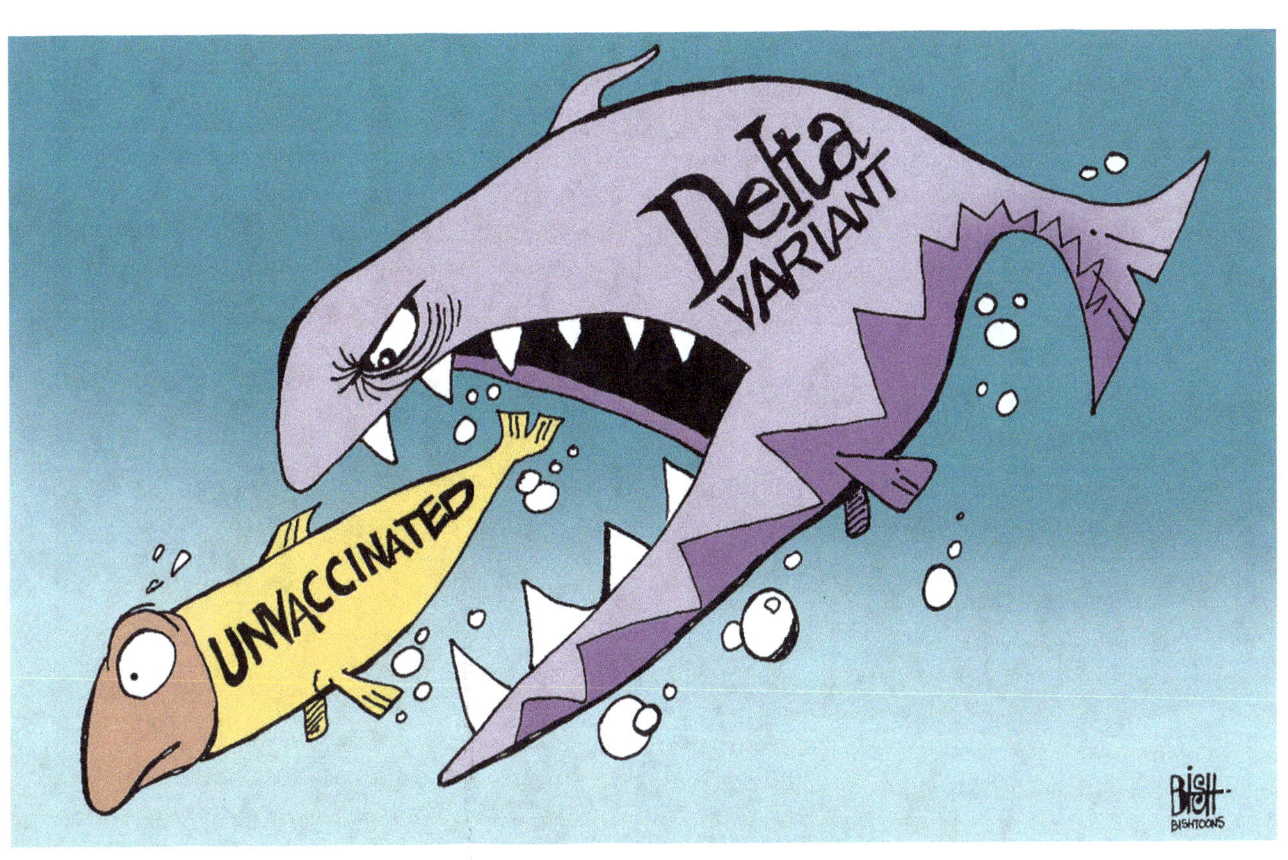

Art by Randy Bish.

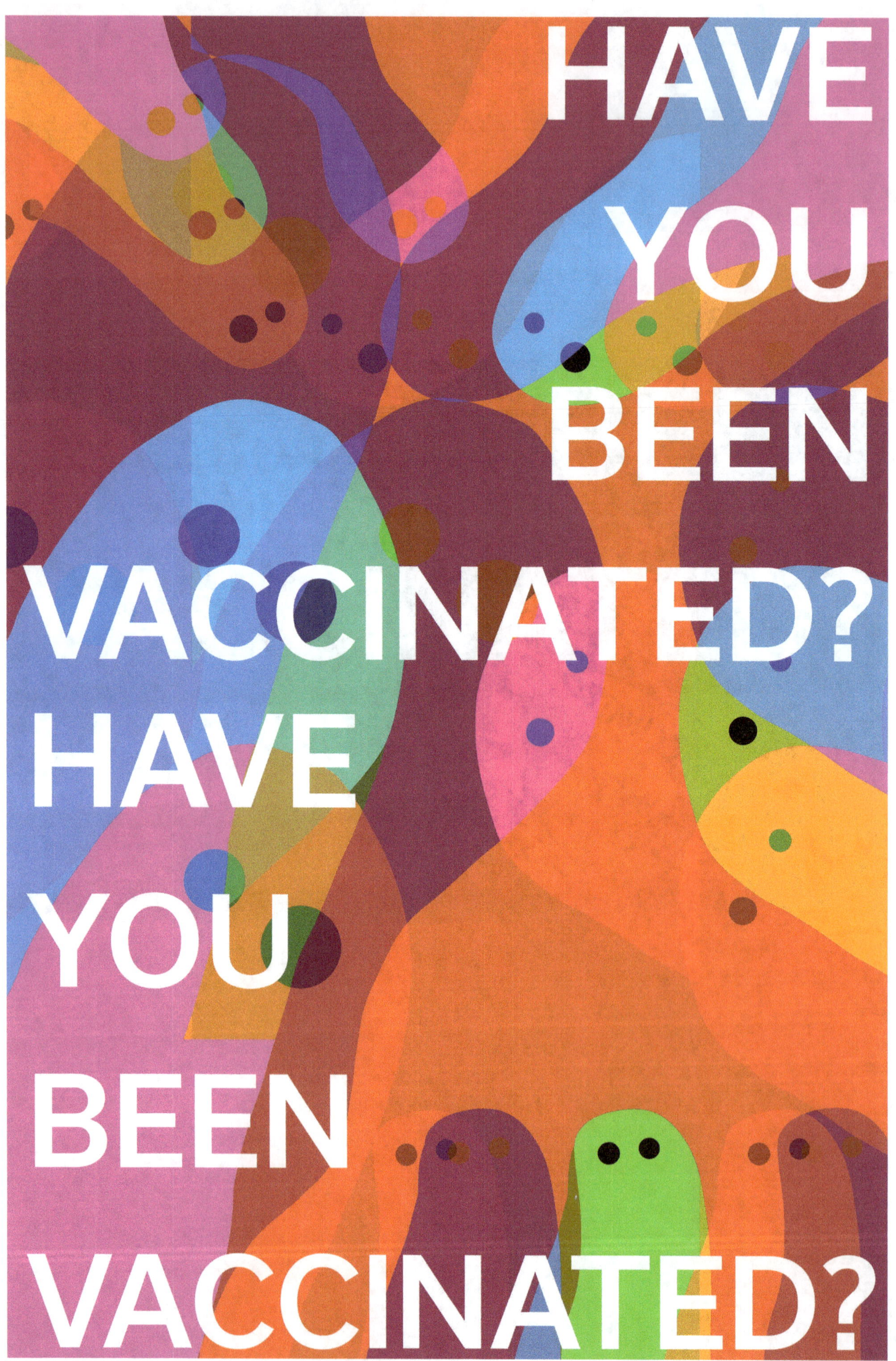

Art by Margaret Elsener.

ACCI

AVE

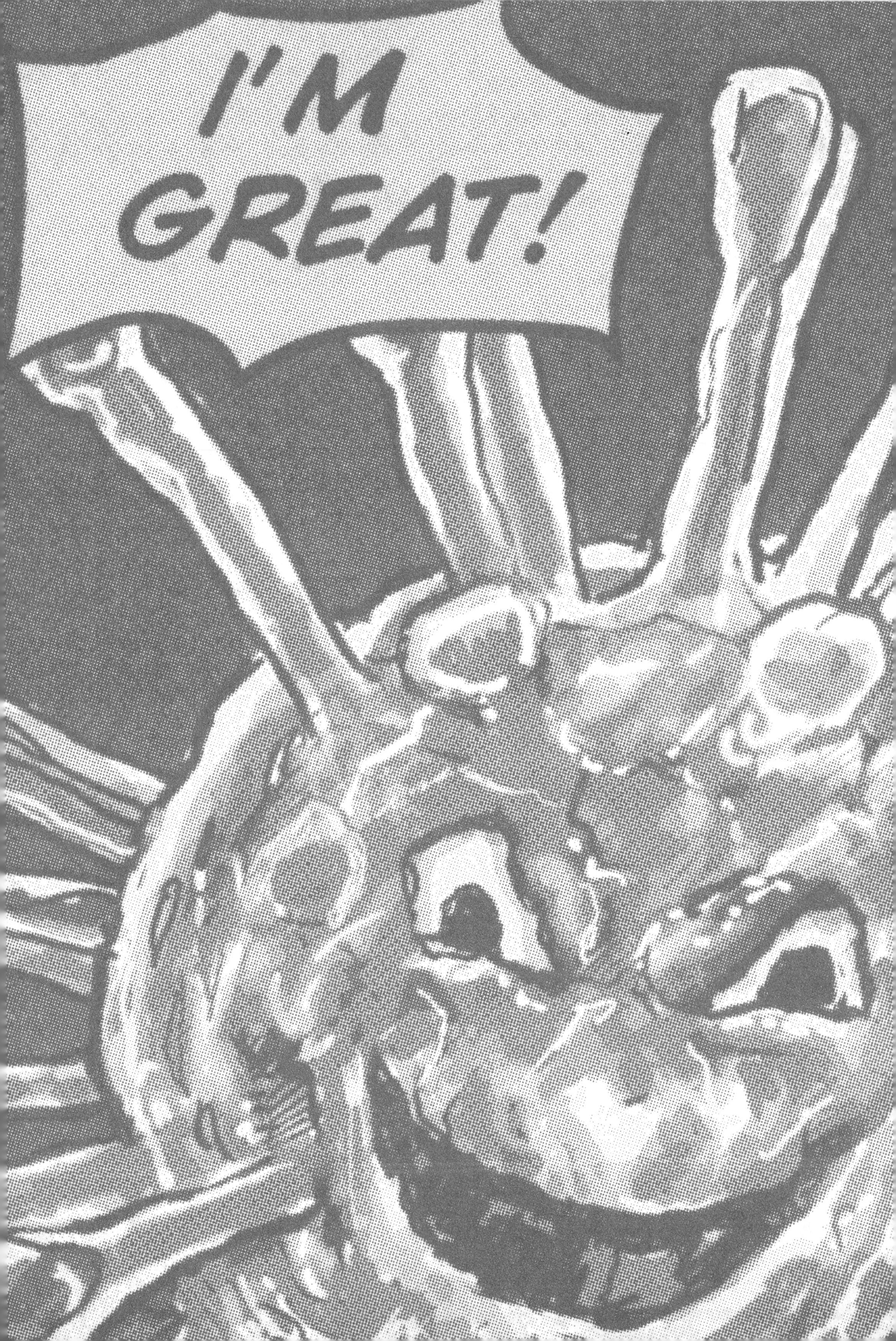
I'M GREAT!

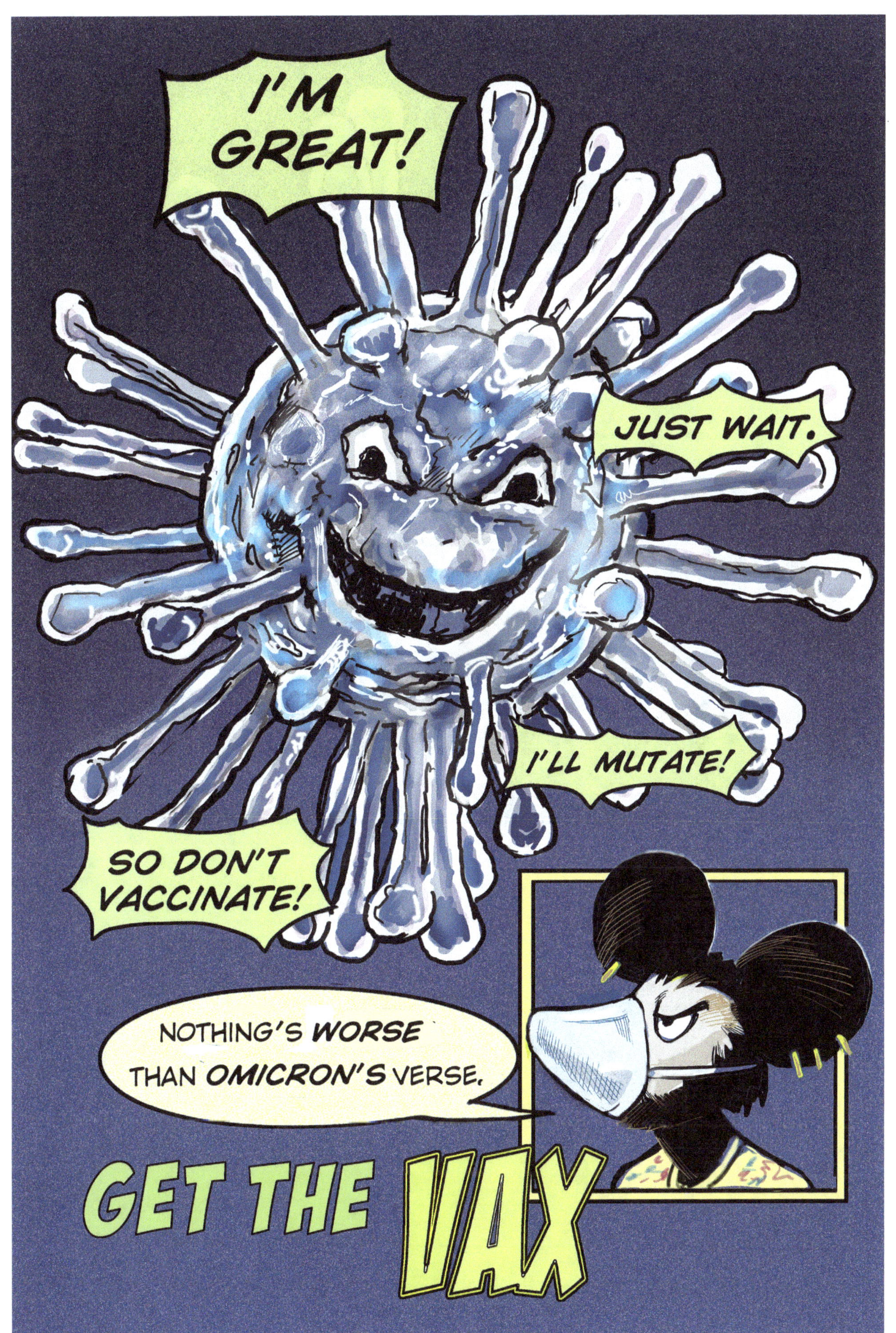

Art by Bob Hall.

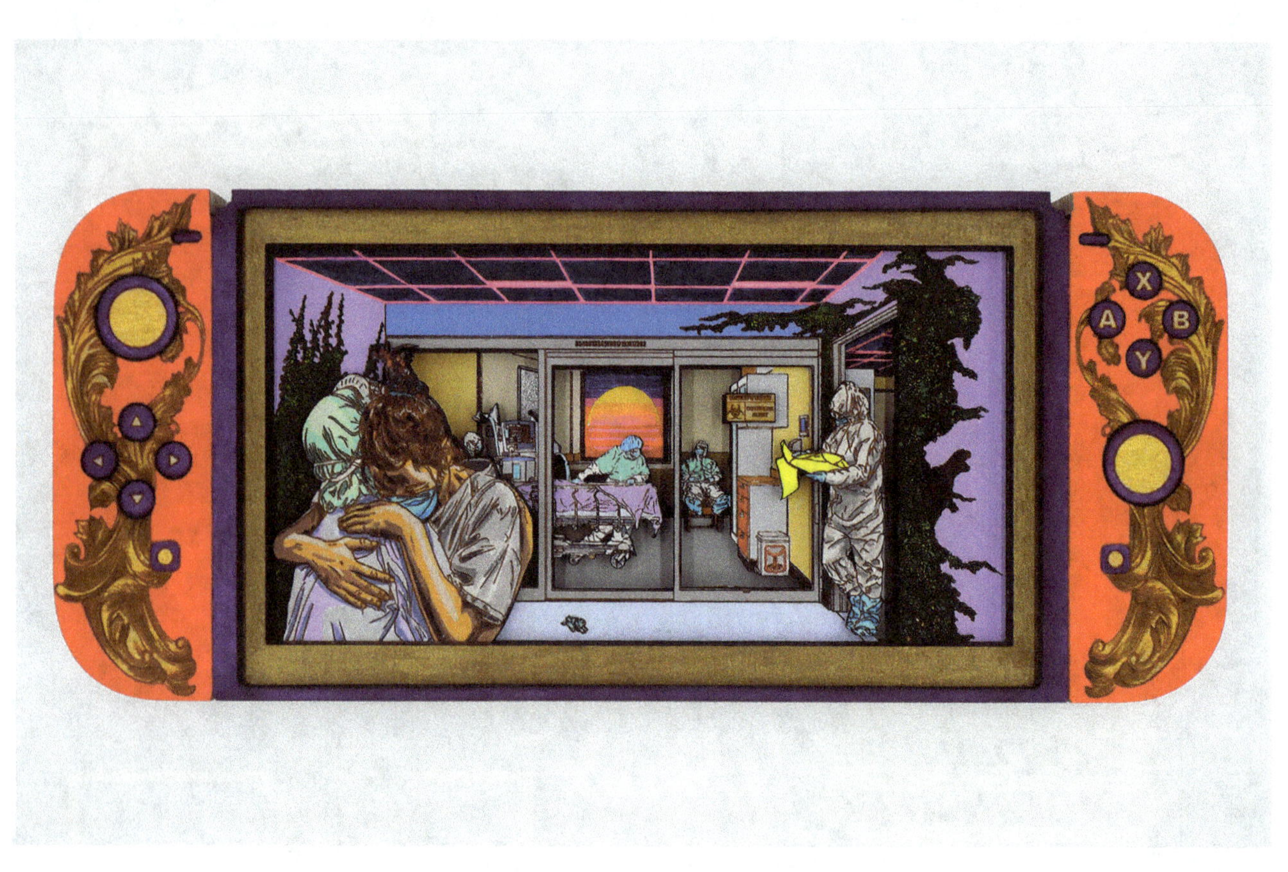

Art by Jave Yoshimoto.

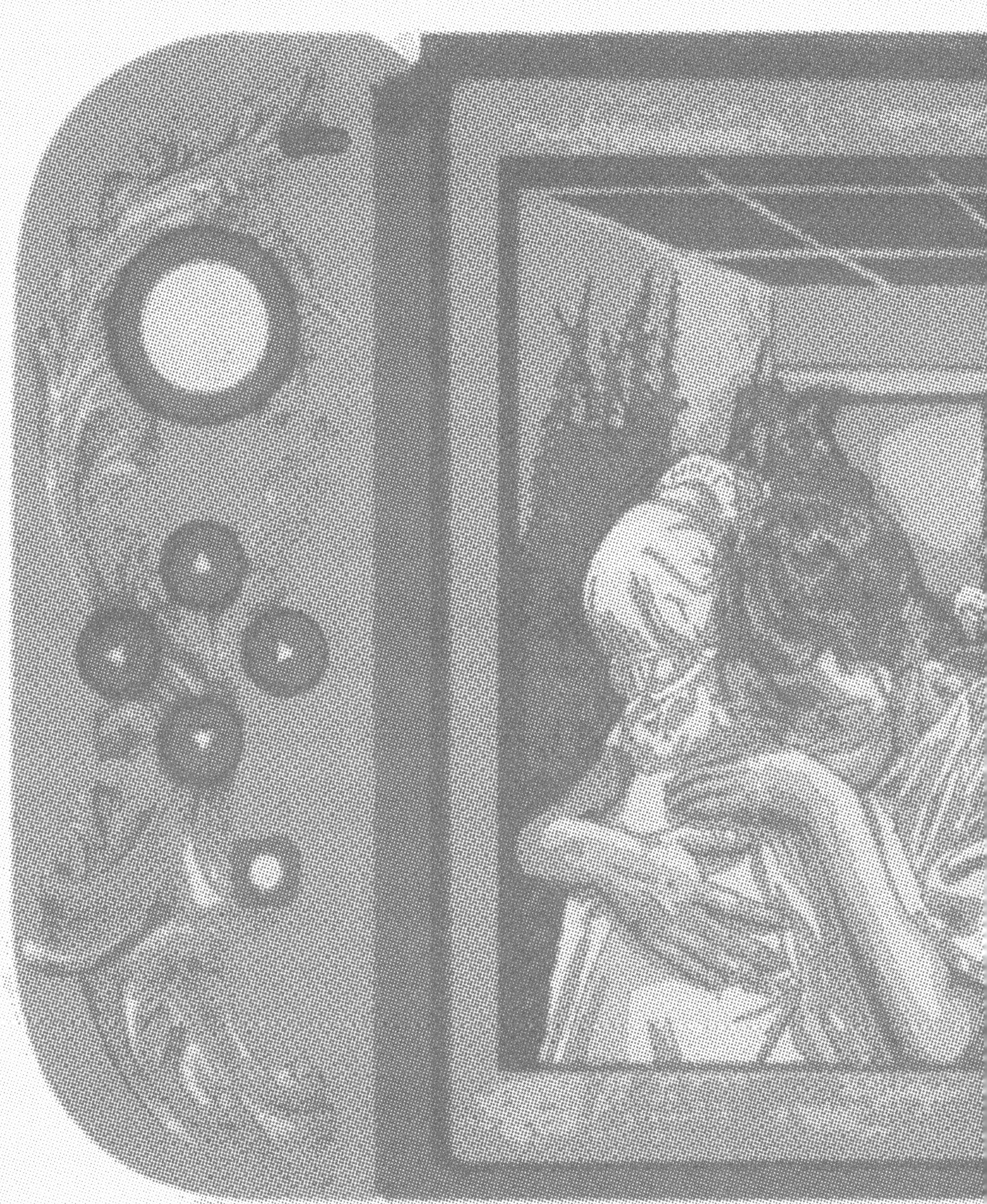

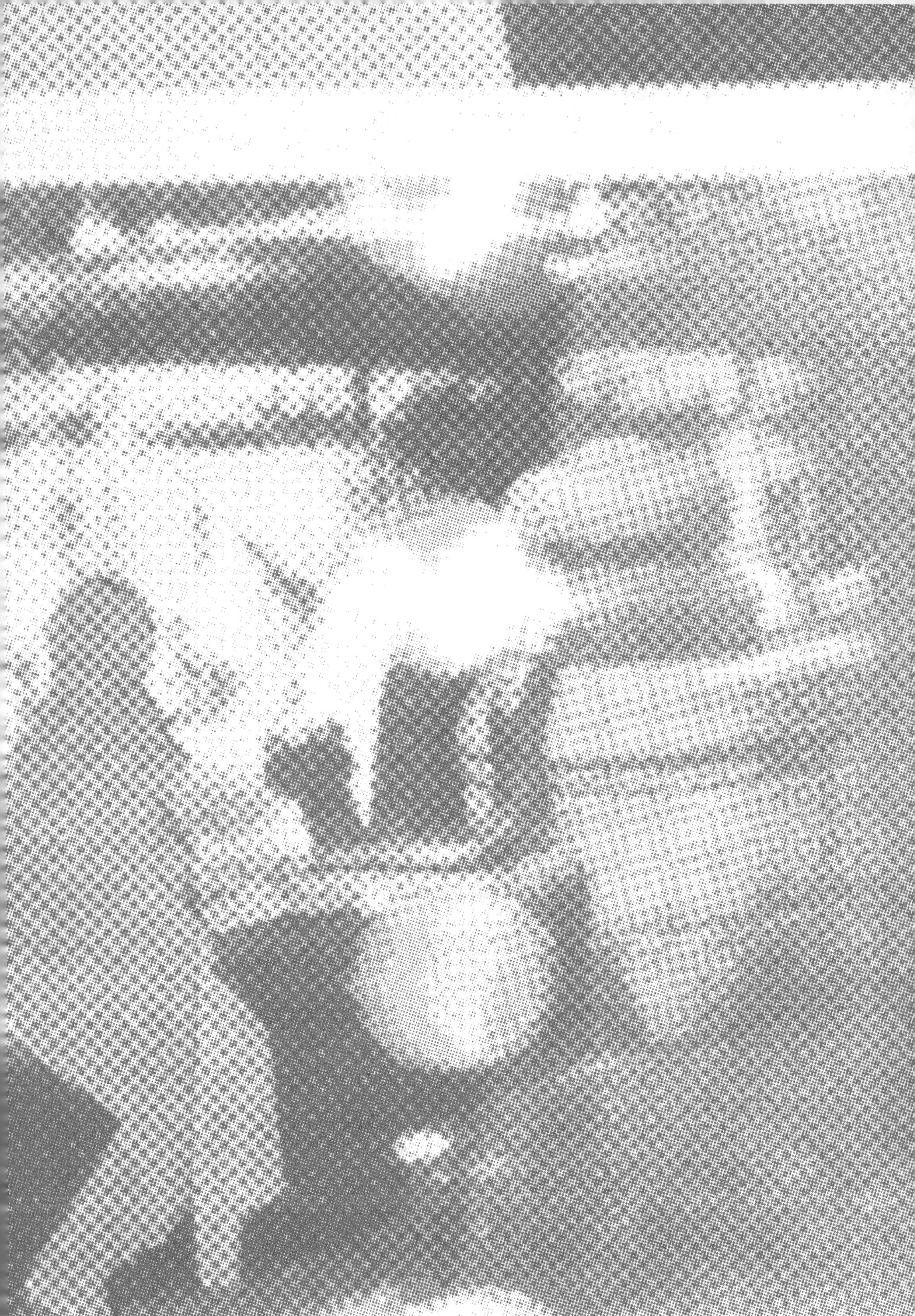

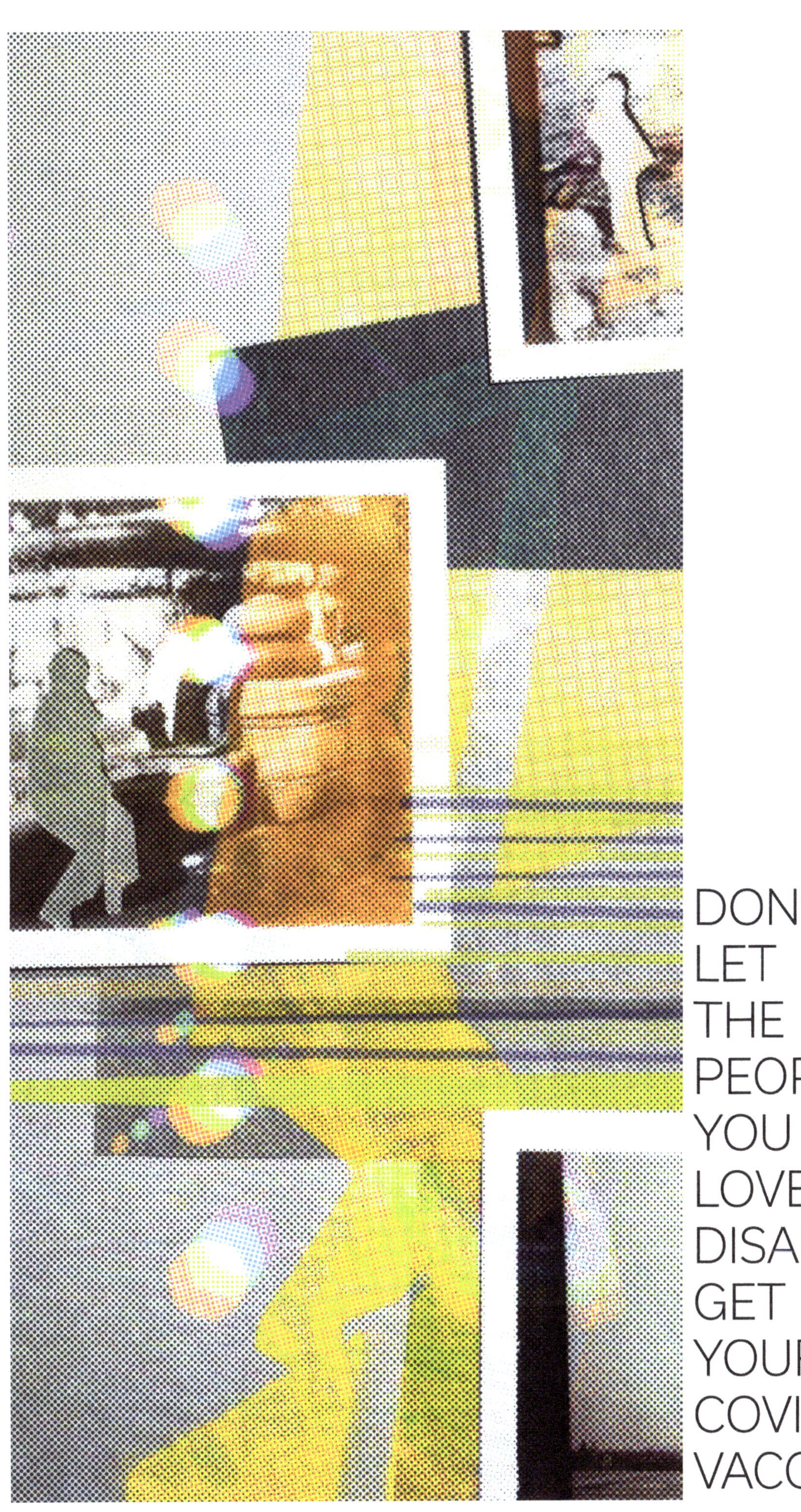

DON'T
LET
THE
PEOPLE
YOU
LOVE
DISAPPEAR.
GET
YOUR
COVID
VACCINE.

Art by Margaret Elsener.

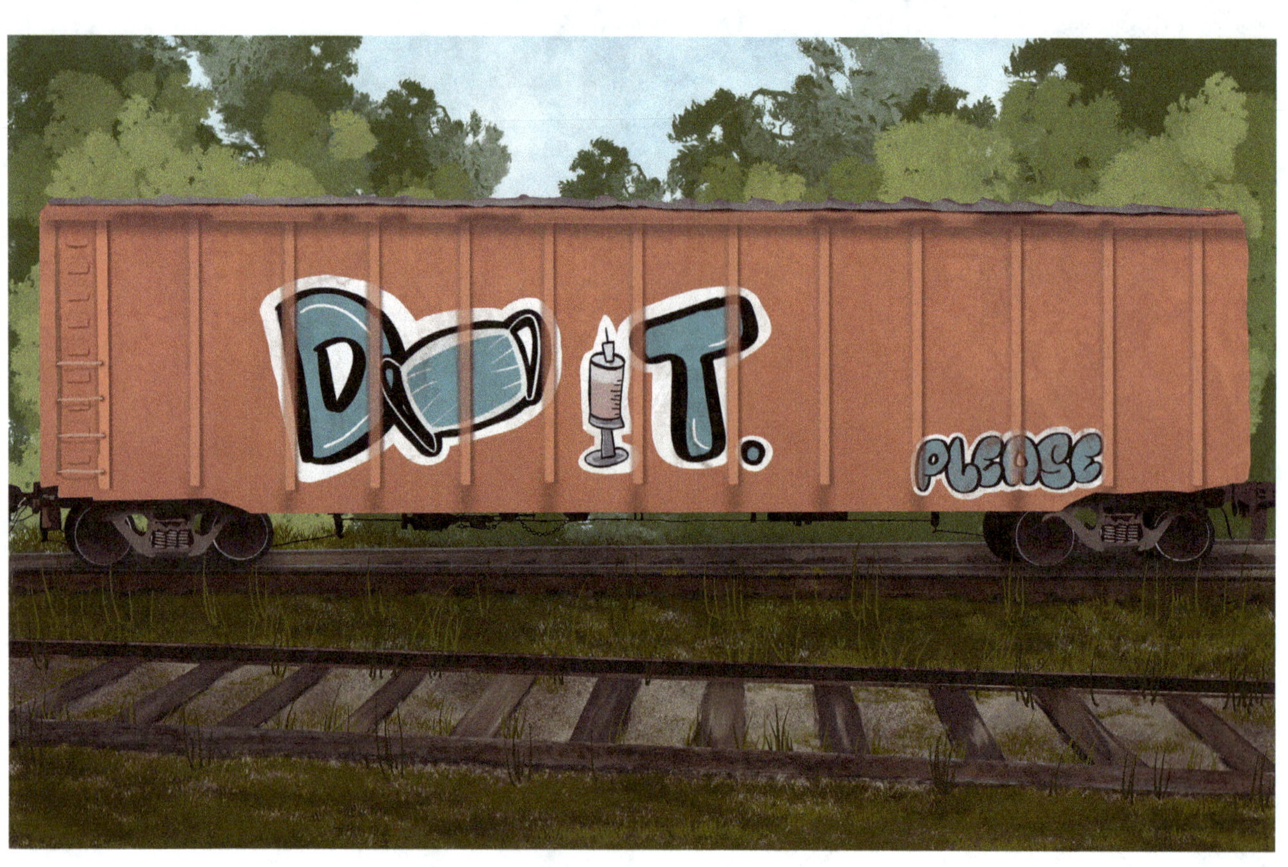

Art by Hayley Jurek and Nikolaus Stevenson.

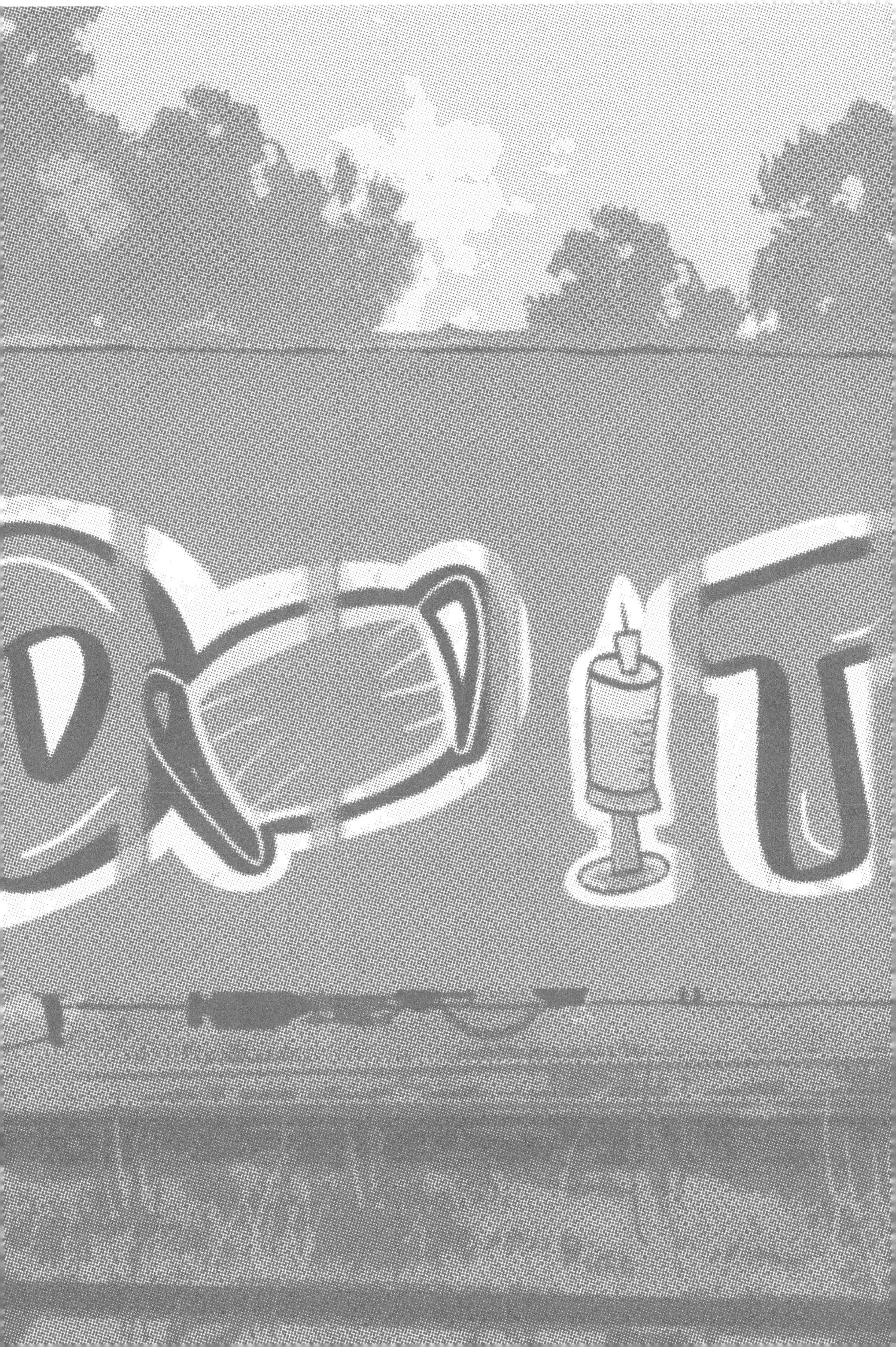

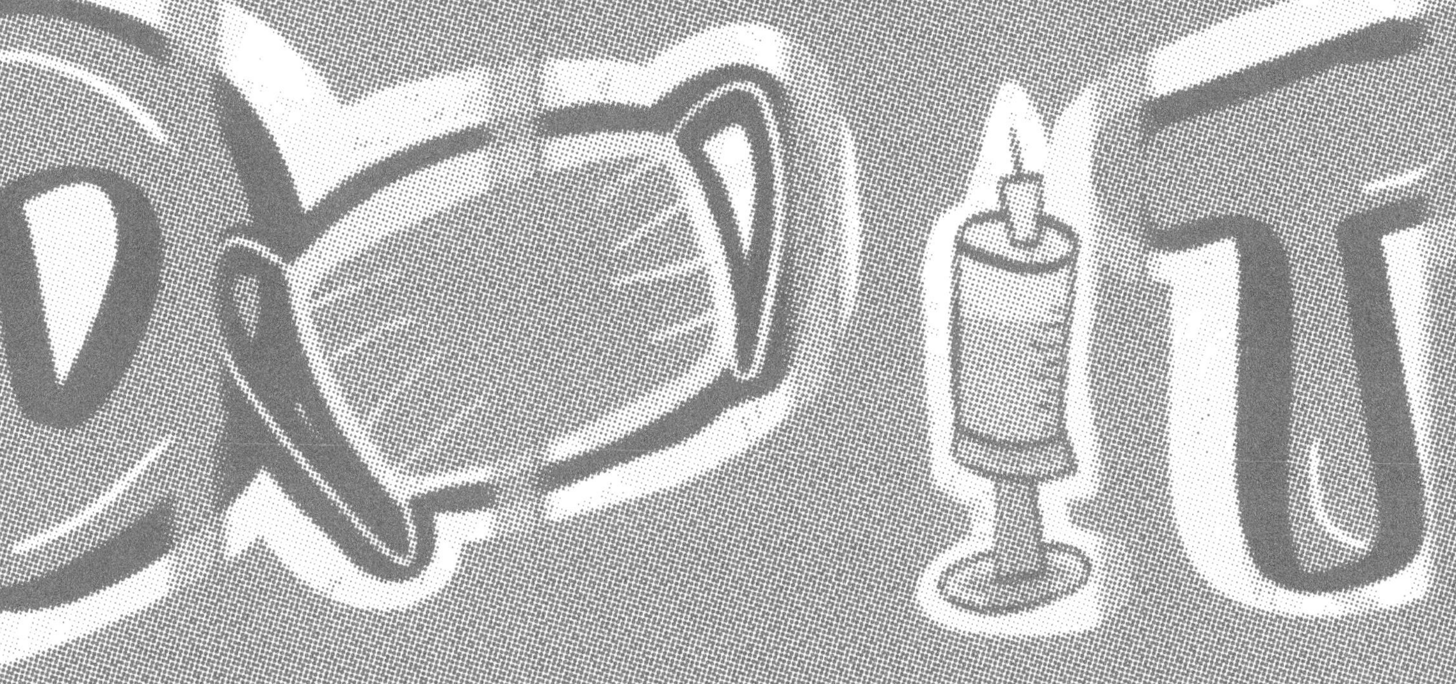

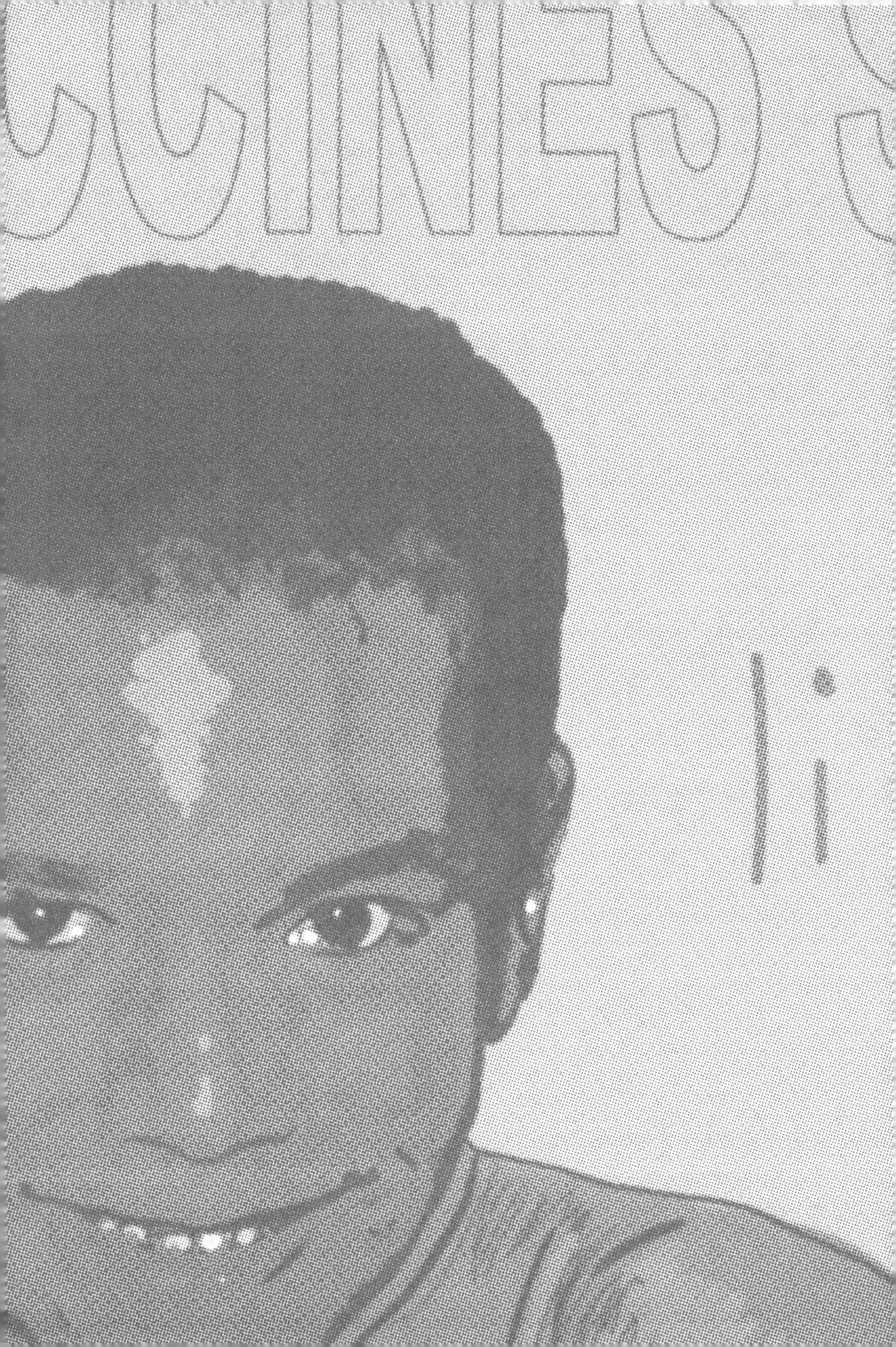

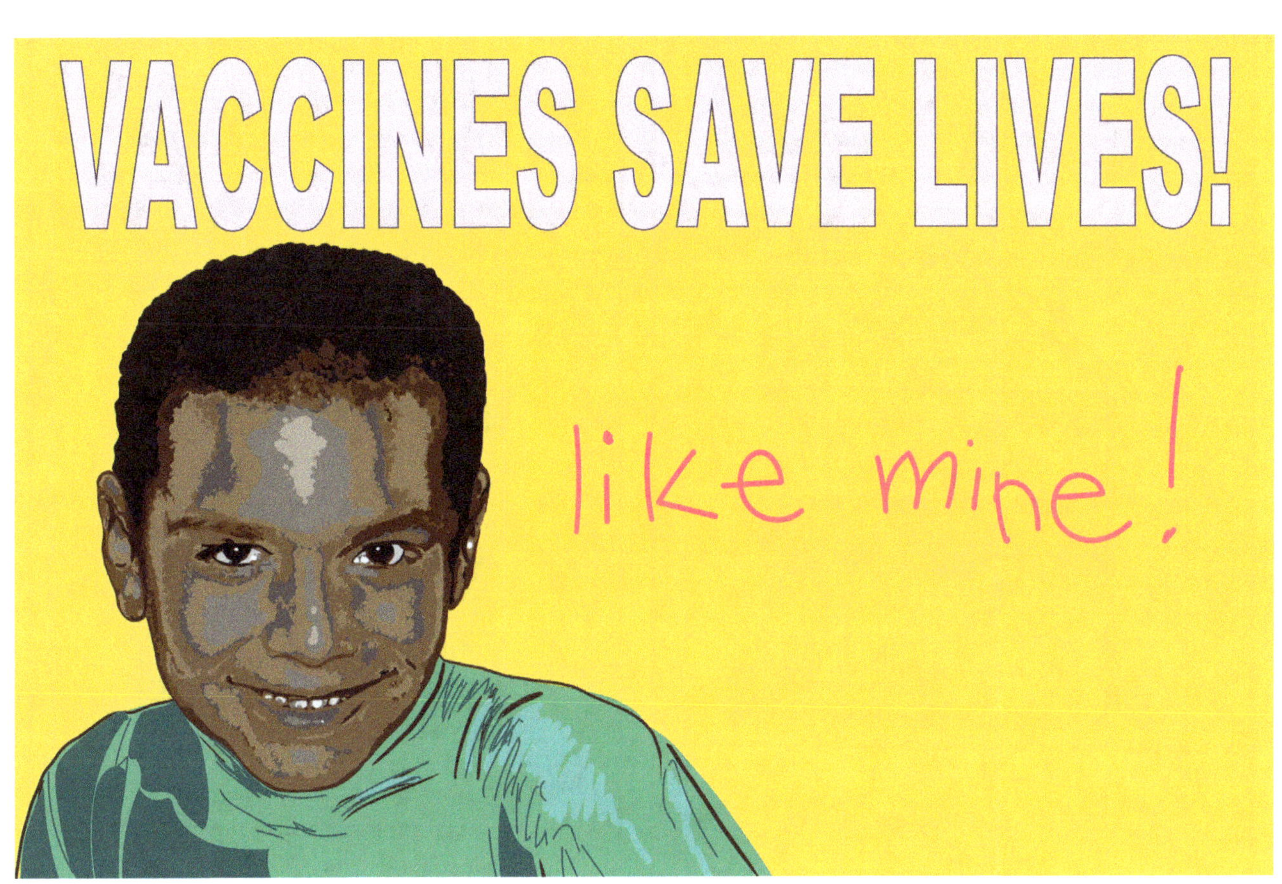

Art by Kerry Eddy.

MARCH 2020

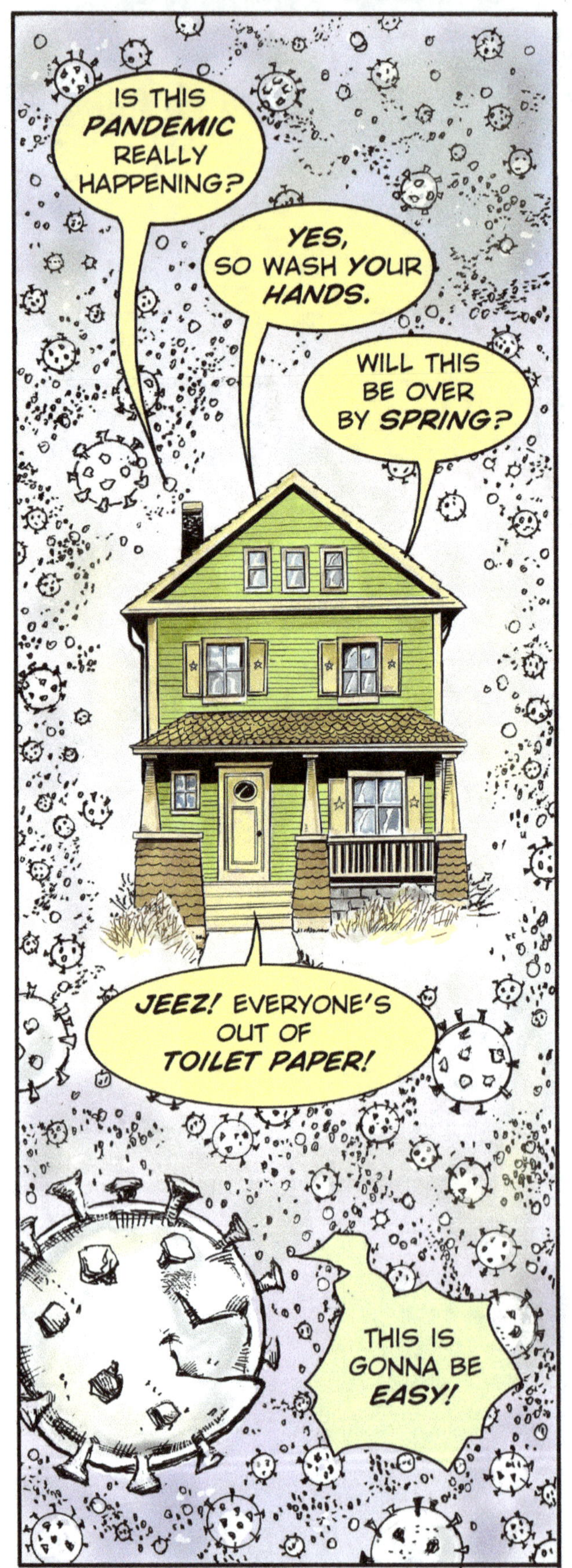

MARCH 2021

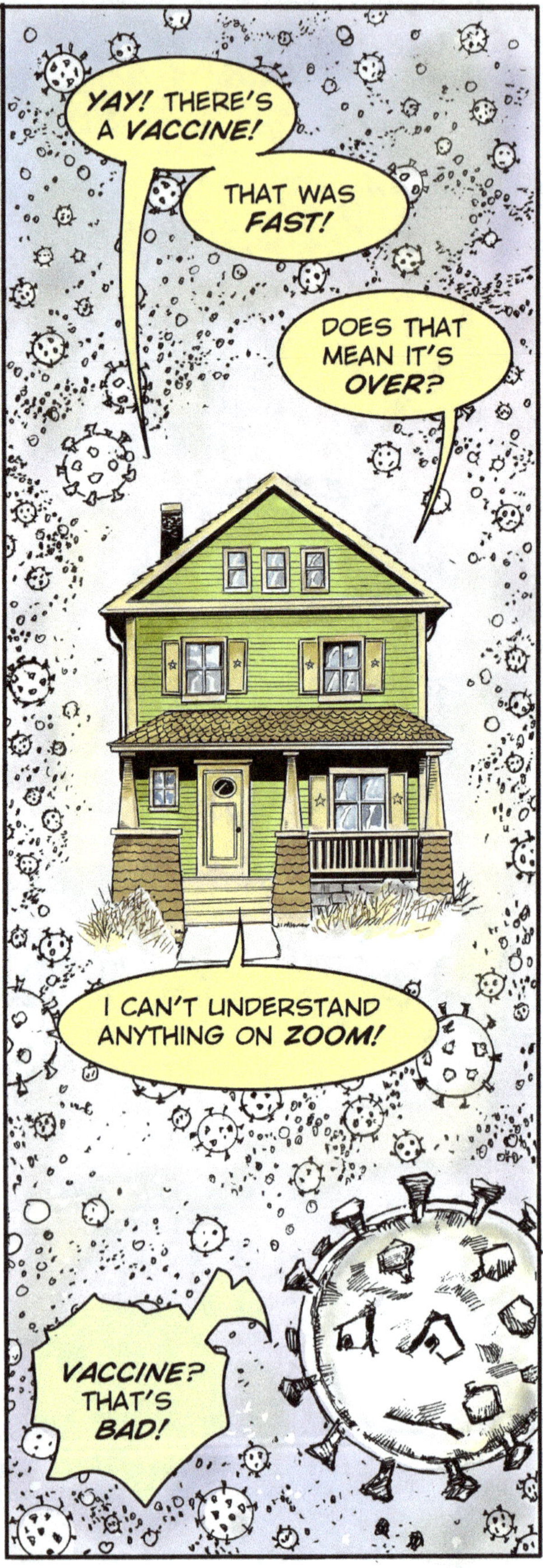

Art by Bob Hall.

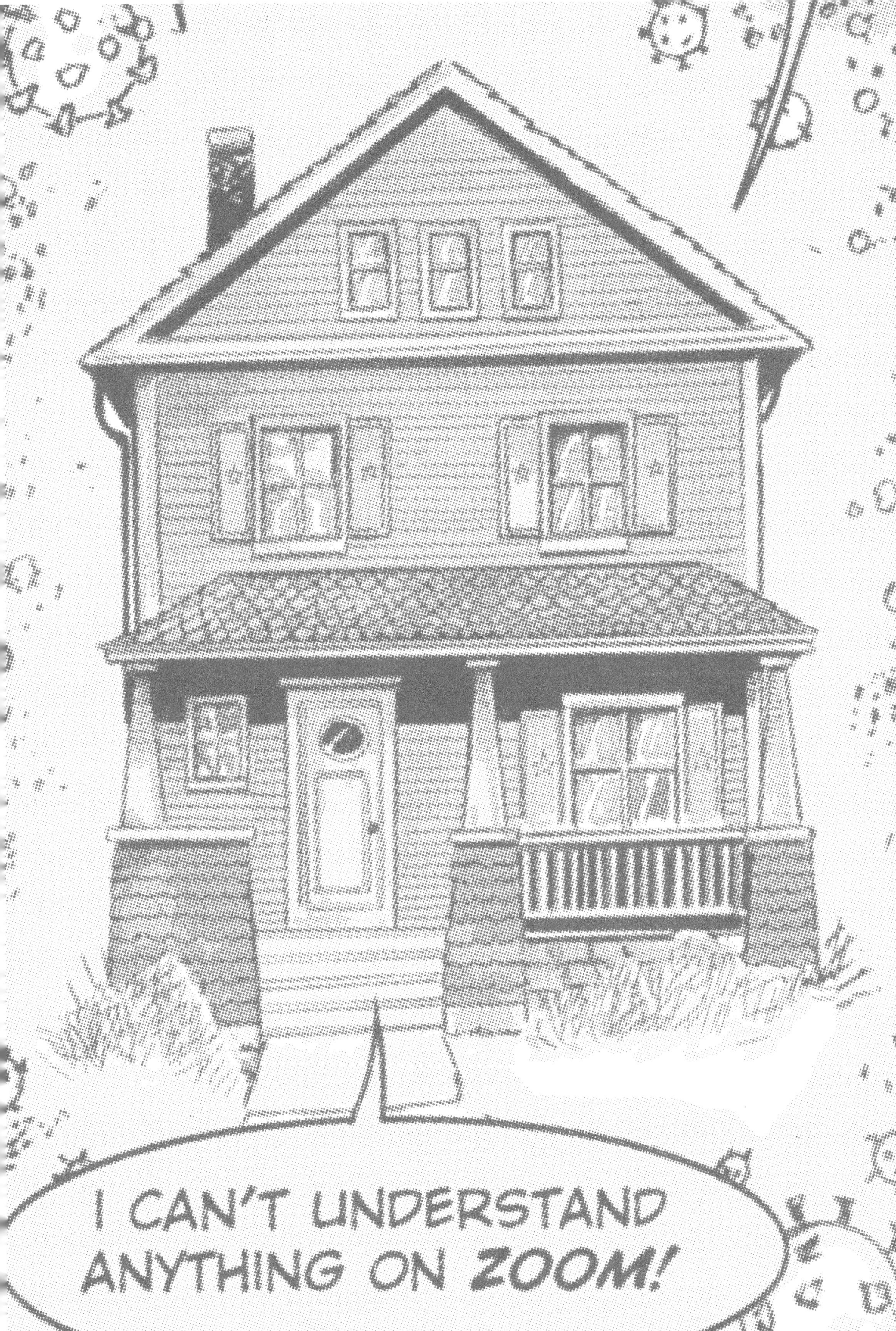
I CAN'T UNDERSTAND
ANYTHING ON ZOOM!

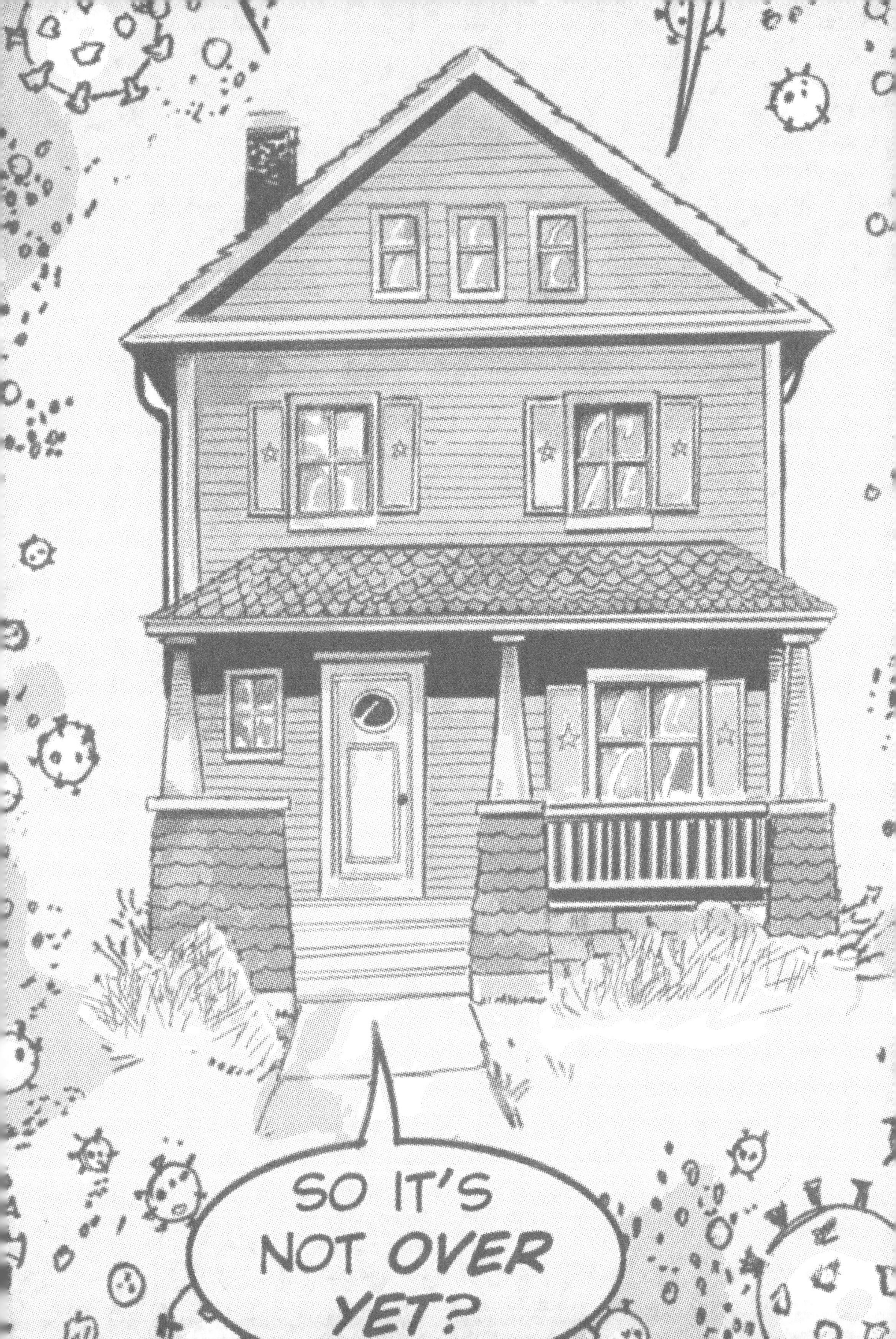
SO IT'S NOT OVER YET?

NOV. 2021

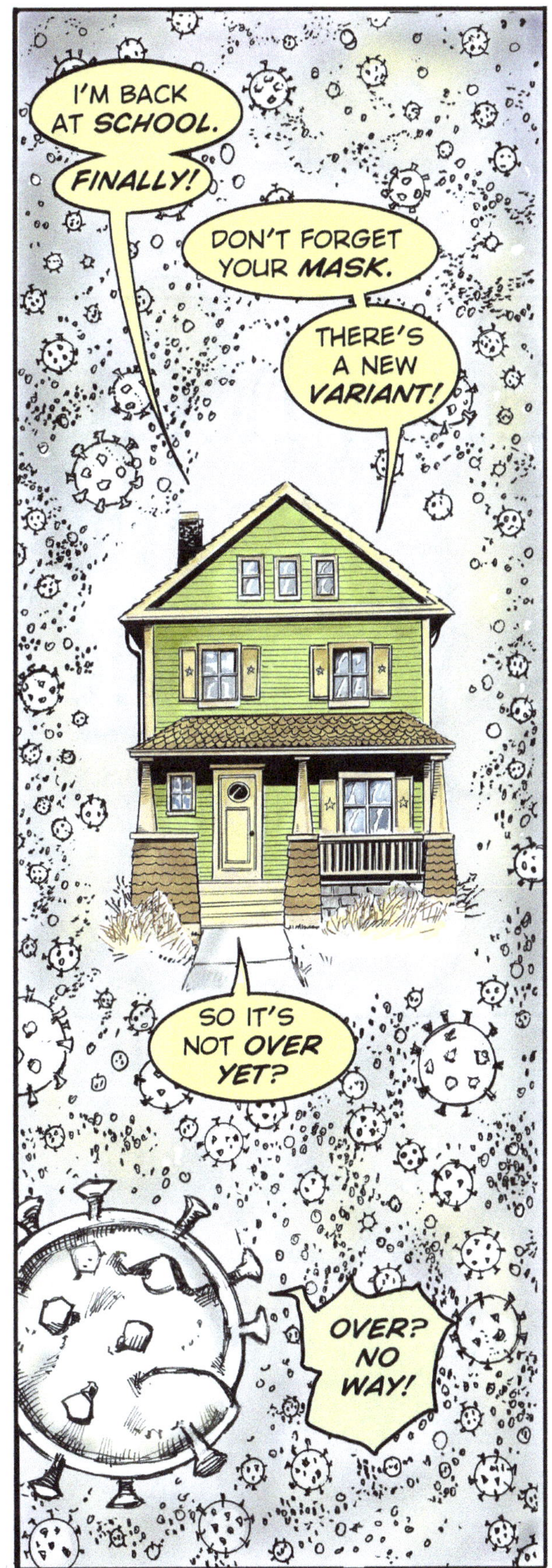

MARCH 2022

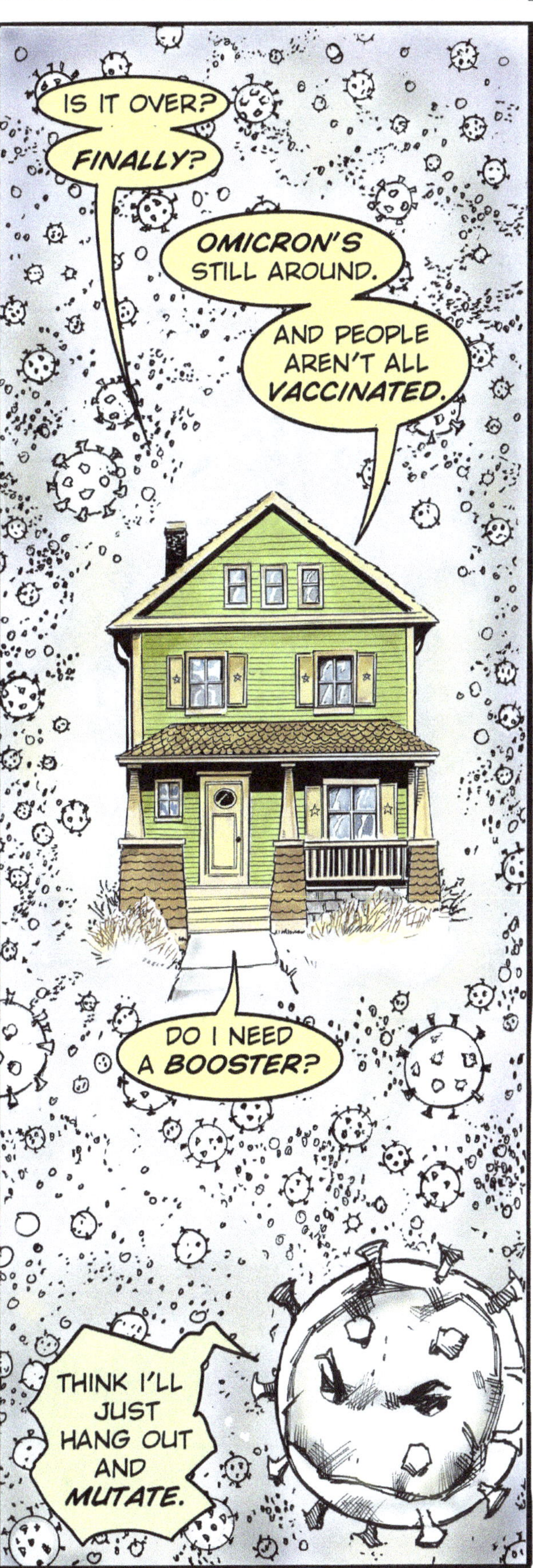

Art by Bob Hall.

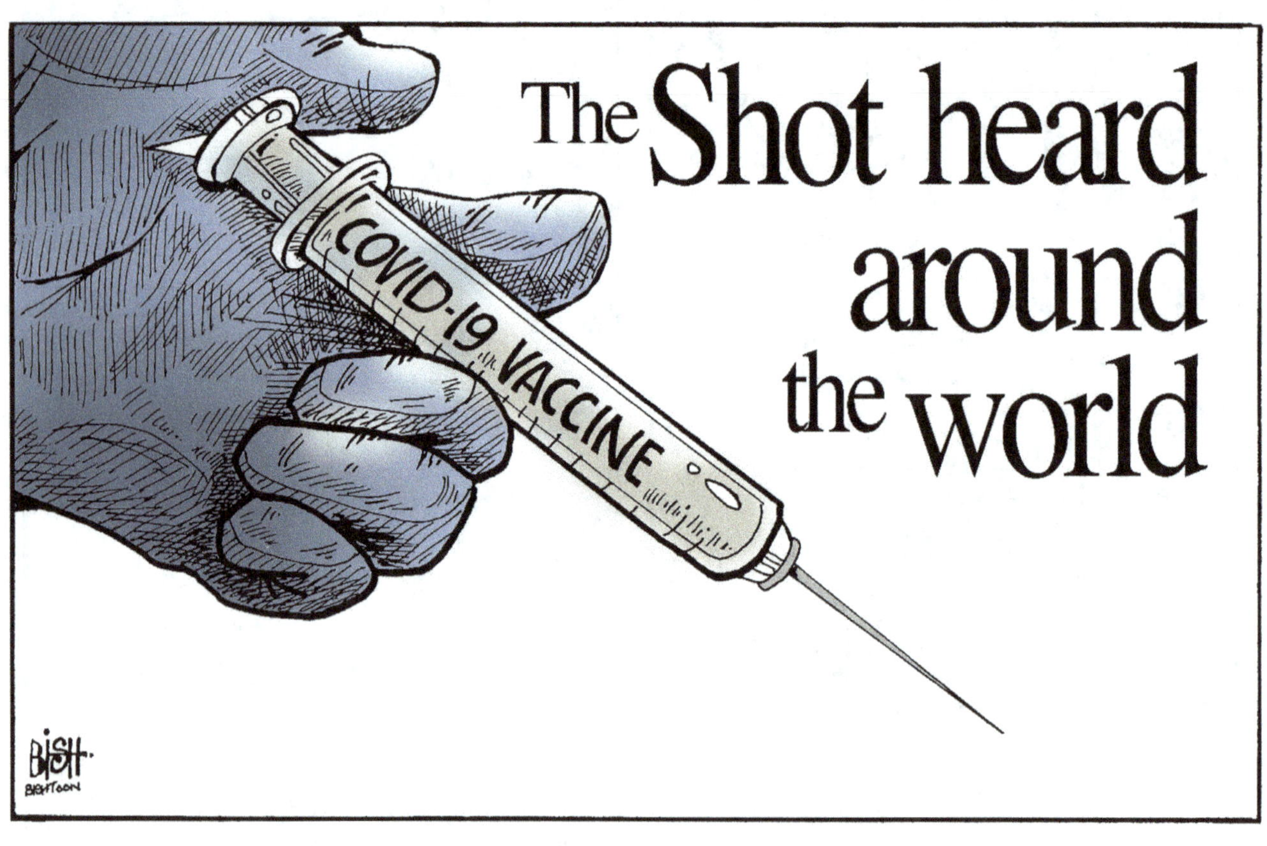

Art by Randy Bish

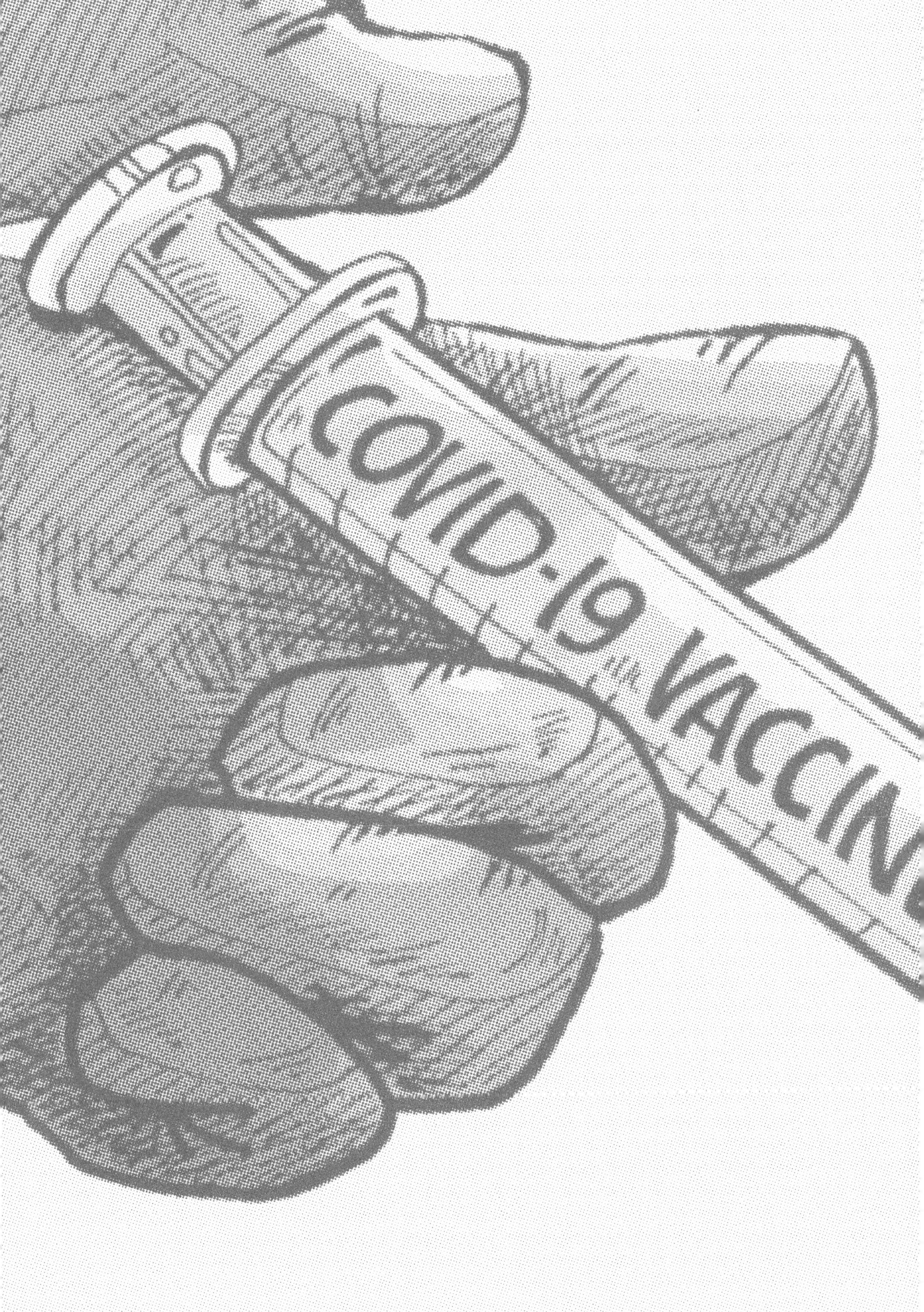
COVID-19 VACCIN

WORLDS OF CONNECTIONS: VACCINE HESITANCY PROJECT TEAM

Judy Diamond, professor, University of Nebraska Libraries, and Curator, University of Nebraska State Museum at Morrill Hall, University of Nebraska–Lincoln

Trish Wonch Hill, research associate professor of sociology, University of Nebraska–Lincoln

Olyvia Kastner, undergraduate research assistant, Worlds of Connections Science Education Partnership Award, University of Nebraska–Lincoln

Meghan Leadabrand, project coordinator, Worlds of Connections Science Education Partnership Award, University of Nebraska–Lincoln

Julia McQuillan, Willa Cather Professor of Sociology, University of Nebraska–Lincoln

Amy N. Spiegel, research associate professor, Methodology and Evaluation Research Core, University of Nebraska–Lincoln

Aaron Sutherlen, associate professor of art, University of Nebraska–Lincoln

Elizabeth VanWormer, One Health coordinator and associate professor of veterinary medicine and biological sciences, University of Nebraska–Lincoln

PROJECT ADVISORS

Judi gaiashkibos, executive director, Nebraska Commission on Indian Affairs

Bob Hall, comic artist, writer, and playwright

St Patrick Reid, assistant professor of pathology and microbiology, University of Nebraska Medical Center

Gregg Wright, professor emeritus, University of Nebraska–Lincoln, and former director of health, Nebraska State Health Department

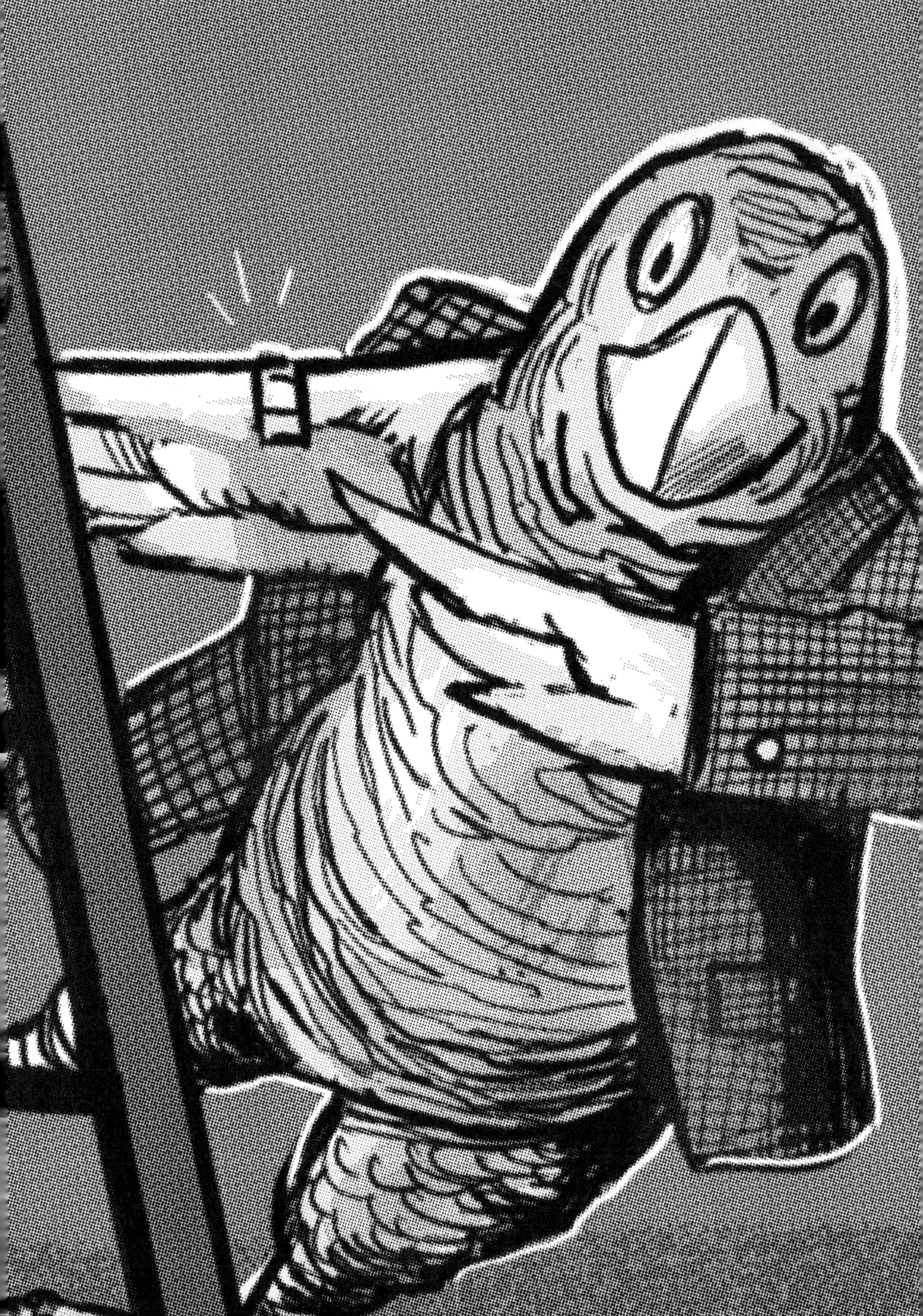

We'd also like to thank . . .

Dr. Tony Beck, program director,
Science Education Partnership Award,
National Institues of Health

Park Middle School Boys and Girls Club

Vanja Bilinac

Joel Brehm

Jane Ferreyra

Kayla Gaertig

Conleigh Hemmer

Nestor Hernandez

Simone Hill

Elizabeth Jardee

Thealouise Lahey

Jaime Long

Sara Mattson

Brecken Obermueller

Henry Payer

Karen Rodriguez

Roxanne Smith

Destiny Spurlock

Elaine Stamper

Penny Thompson

Adam Wong

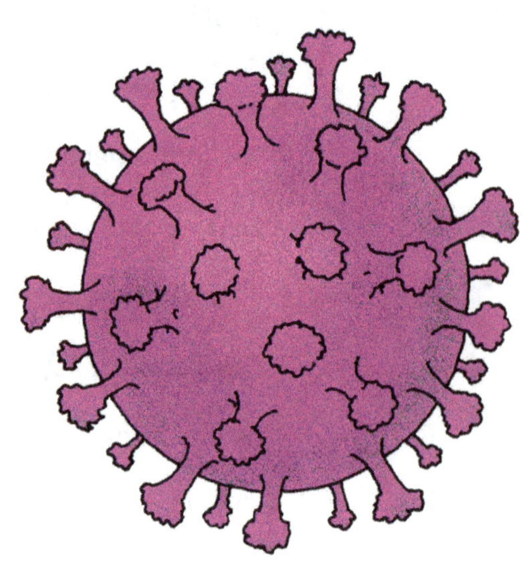

ABOUT THE CONTRIBUTING ARTISTS

Rachel Claire Balter is a graphic designer and digital artist from Chicago, Illinois. In her spare time, she collects antique teacups.

Thane Benson is an independent comic writer and artist best known for the infernal murder mystery graphic novel *Burnt* and the ongoing *Quick the Clockwork Knight* series. Originally from New York, Thane lives in Denver, Colorado.

Randy Bish, born in Kittanning, Pennsylvania, has been drawing editorial cartoons for newspapers since the early 1980s. His work may be found in museums and on refrigerator doors around the world.

Katie Bradshaw grew up in the Chicago area and now lives in Wyobraska. She expresses herself in various art forms including blogs, zines, collages, stained glass pieces, and gingerbread structures.

Heinzy Cruz is a writer, penciler and musician based in Zapopan, Mexico. They are the creator of the comic *The Circle of Aquarious* and the guitar player of the band Human Eve.

Hector Curriel is a contemporary visual artist and storyteller who lives and works in Sioux Falls, South Dakota. A native of Lima, Peru, his variety of art production includes fine art, book illustration, and cartooning. His distinctive personal composition style emanates different stages of the human spirit.

Ben Darling creates art in Sidney, Nebraska, and is involved with art encouragement and education privately and through the Nebraska Arts Council. Working in painting, relief printmaking, and drawing, he explores a wide range of subjects and topics, which have wonderfully tangential areas of study: weather, gardening, botany, archeology, geology, and social activism.

Nicholas Deason is a research biologist with an interest in science communication. He is based in San Diego, California.

Kerry Eddy is an artist, musician, designer, illustrator, and multimedia practitioner. She enjoys poodle worship, cat petting, pixel manipulation, pushing watery pigments around on paper, making indelible marks, creating vibes, plucking strings, screaming quietly, experimenting with video, creating atmospheres, and making melodic and rhythmic noises. She is from Lincoln, Nebraska.

Margaret Elsener is an artist and art educator in Lincoln, Nebraska. She oscillates between the worlds of being the Jane-of-all-trades that art education requires, creating her own work, collecting tropical house plants, and visiting as many state and national parks as she can in this lifetime.

Paul Fell has been a freelance editorial cartoonist/illustrator since 1992 and has also been a high school art teacher, a college art professor, and newspaper editorial cartoonist. He is the author and co-author of several cartoon books, and his editorial cartoons are syndicated by Artizans.com and CartoonStock.com.

David L. Felley is a retired carpenter and wildlife biologist living and avoiding work in eastern Oregon with his wife and two cats. David is a dabbler in many things, which until recently didn't include watercolor.

Bob Hall is a comic artist, writer, playwright, and theatrical director known for his work with Marvel Comics. He has collaborated with National Institutes of Health–and National Science Foundation–funded teams at the University of Nebraska on graphic stories and essays, including *C'RONA Pandemic Comics* (University of Nebraska Press 2021) and *Carnival of Contagion* (University of Nebraska Press 2017). He lives in Lincoln, Nebraska.

Hayley Jurek is the communication and design specialist for the STEM TRAIL Center at the University of Nebraska–Omaha. On weekends you can find her photographing kids and families or baking whatever sweet treat popped up on her Pinterest page that week.

Justin Kemerling is an independent designer, activist, and collaborator living in Omaha, Nebraska, focused on making it beautiful, moving people to action, and getting good things done.

Abbey Krienke, DDS, grew up in Pierce, Nebraska, and currently resides in Lincoln. Apart from work, she enjoys visiting local coffee shops, art galleries, and parks; working in the garden; and spending time with her husband and three children.

Stephen Lahey is a professor who studies medieval theology at the University of Nebraska–Lincoln and a priest in the Episcopal Church of the United States. A U.S. Navy veteran, he enthusiastically paints and draws whenever possible.

Anna Lindstrom is a young artist from Broken Bow, Nebraska.

Malia McCreight enjoys art, animals, and Pokémon.

Yihang Meng is a young artist from China who is now studying at the University of Nebraska–Lincoln.

Eric Morris is a speculative writer and multi-media artist from Bellevue, Nebraska. They are an amateur bookmaker, future novelist, certified sweet tooth, and professional overthinker.

Katie Nieland is a Great Plains artist living in Lincoln, Nebraska, whose work focuses on exploring the natural world. She is a sunny optimist fueled by curiosity, iced coffee, and a passion to share what is good.

Henry Payer is a Ho-Chunk multidisciplinary artist. He has exhibited his work at many locations including Rapid City, South Dakota; Minneapolis, Minnesota; Kansas City, Missouri; and Madison, Wisconsin. He has taught art and art history, earned multiple awards and honors, and was the 2018 Elizabeth Rubendall Artist in Residence at the University of Nebraska–Lincoln's Great Plains Art Museum.

Natalie Pulte, age 9, is a student and loves all things art. She resides in Papillion, Nebraska, with her family.

Nikolaus Stevenson is currently based in Omaha, Nebraska. He loves the outdoors and spending time with his family and dogs.

Pawl Tisdale was born in Lincoln, Nebraska, Earth. He is a graphic designer and cartoonist of a biannual comic book called *Burnt Cookies*. He finds creative inspiration from people-watching and daily tales of the mundane.

Janet Walters of Lincoln, Nebraska, and her son, photographer Benjamin Walters of Ithaca, New York, combined artistic forces for their submission to the Vaccinate project. Drawing on the knowledge that people love dogs and dogs love their humans, Janet used a photo by Benjamin to create a graphic image that would connect with those humans and provoke them to consider vaccination against COVID-19

William Wells, 76, is a designer in California. A graduate of the Art Center in Los Angeles, he has over forty years' experience in the design of permanent museum exhibitions, products, commercial interiors, and the design and illustration of education publications. He lives in Marin County with his wife, a children's book author. He mostly gets around on a bike and, when available, a sailboat.

Jave Yoshimoto is an Omaha-based visual artist and art professor at the University of Nebraska–Omaha. He travels to collect stories from a variety of places and people to inspire his art compositions. Jave is also a competitive axe thrower who competed in the World Axe Throwing Championships in 2020 and 2021. He has received awards for his art, including craftsman of the year for custom axe designs.

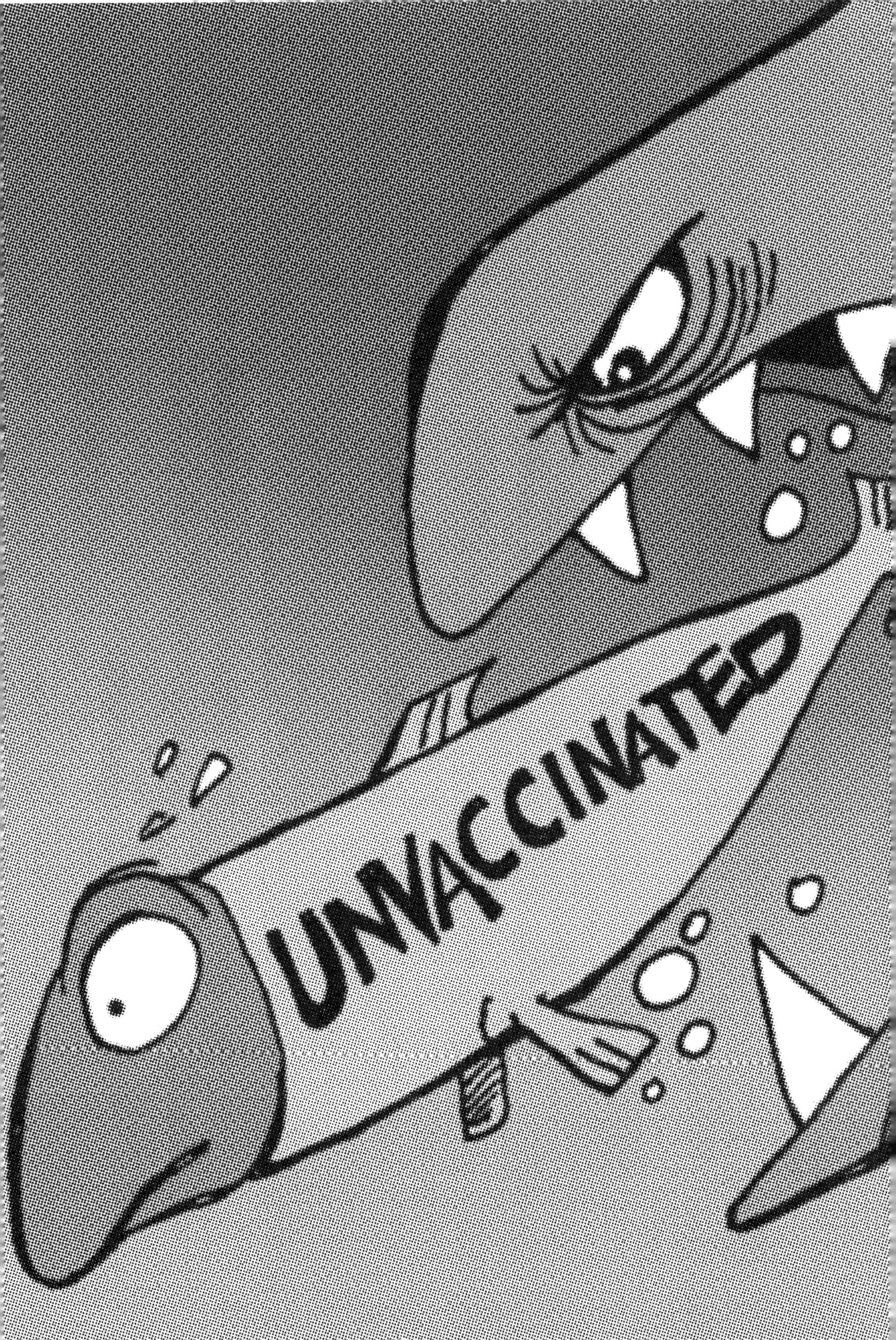
UNVACCINATED

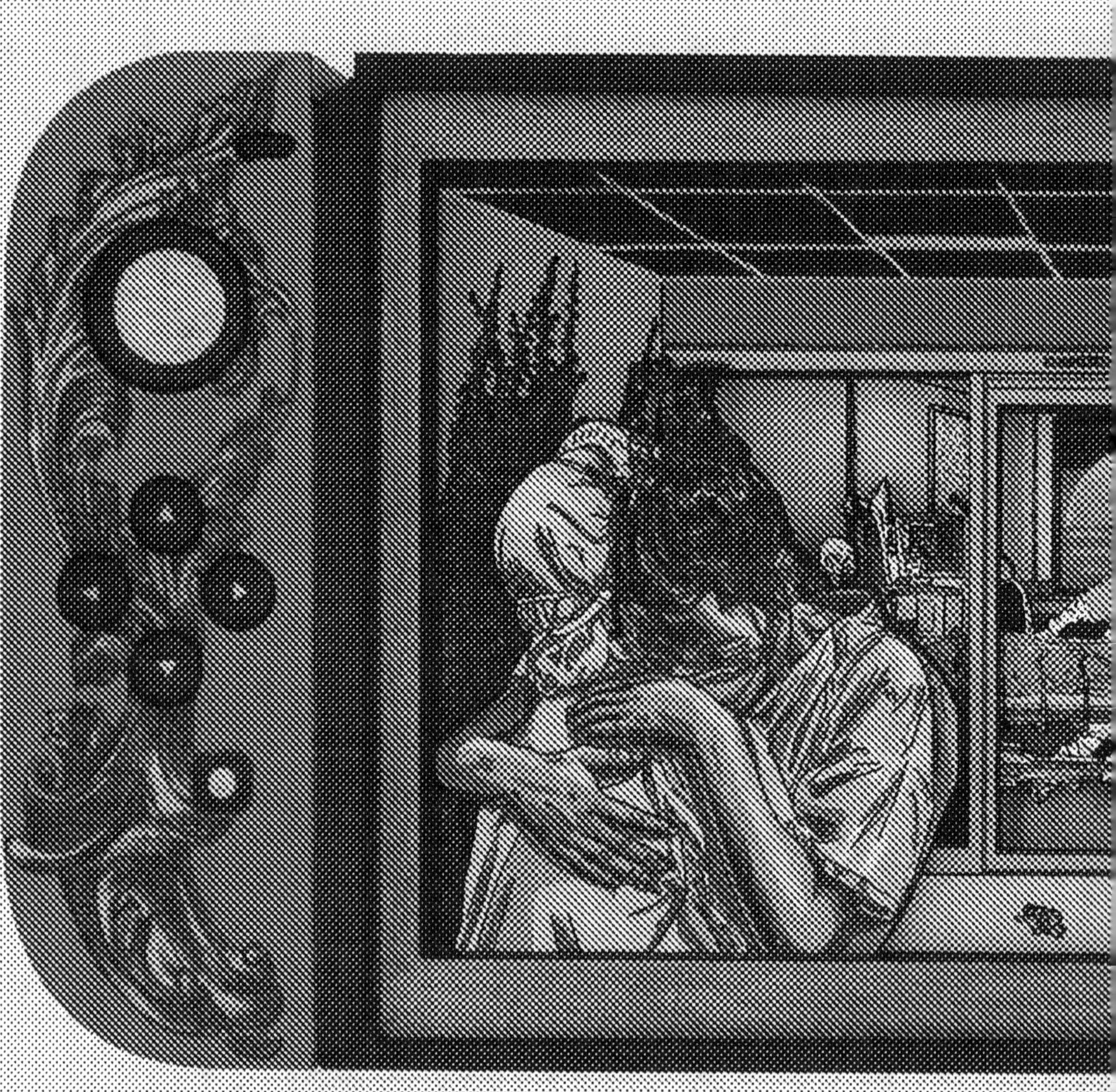

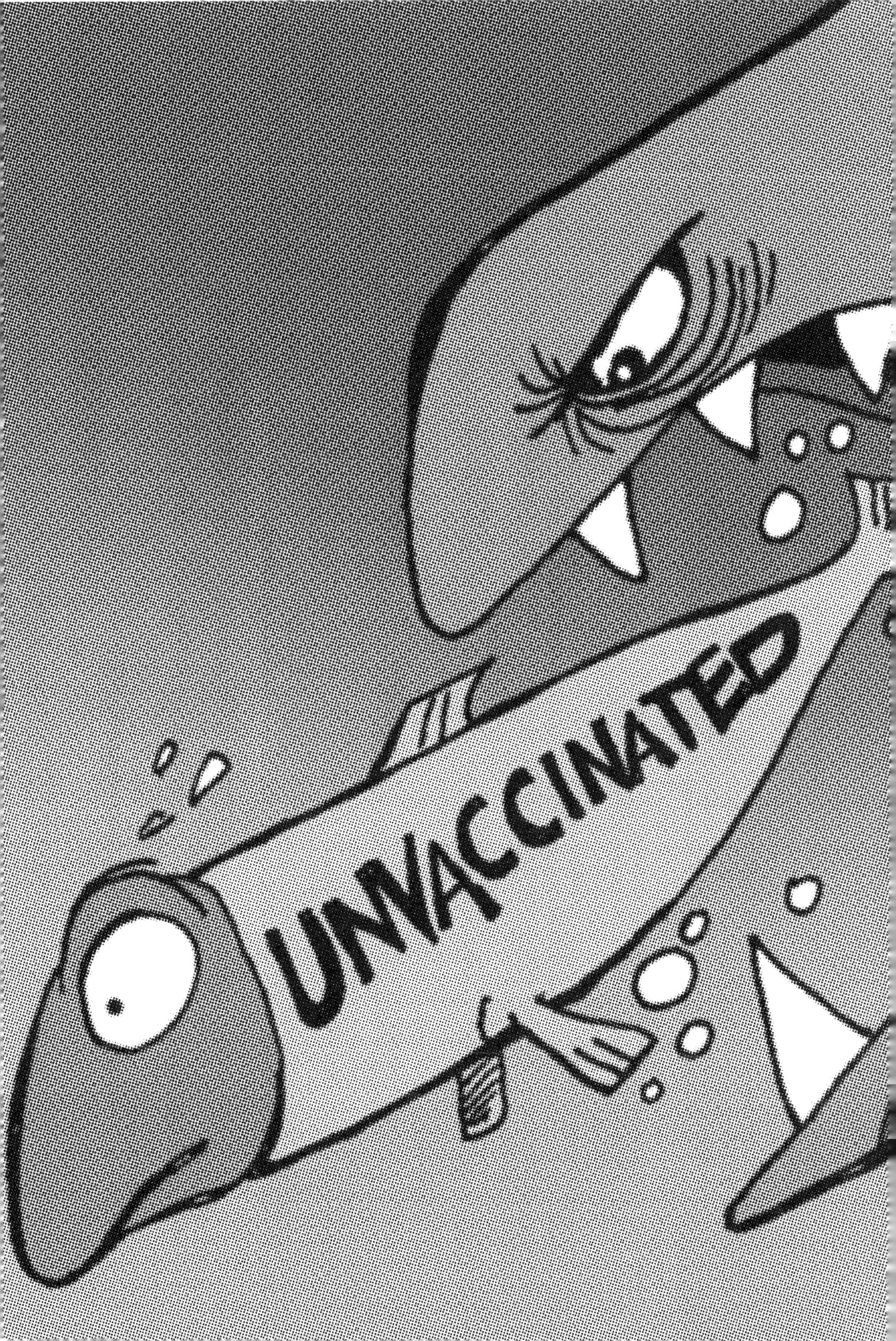
UNVACCINATED

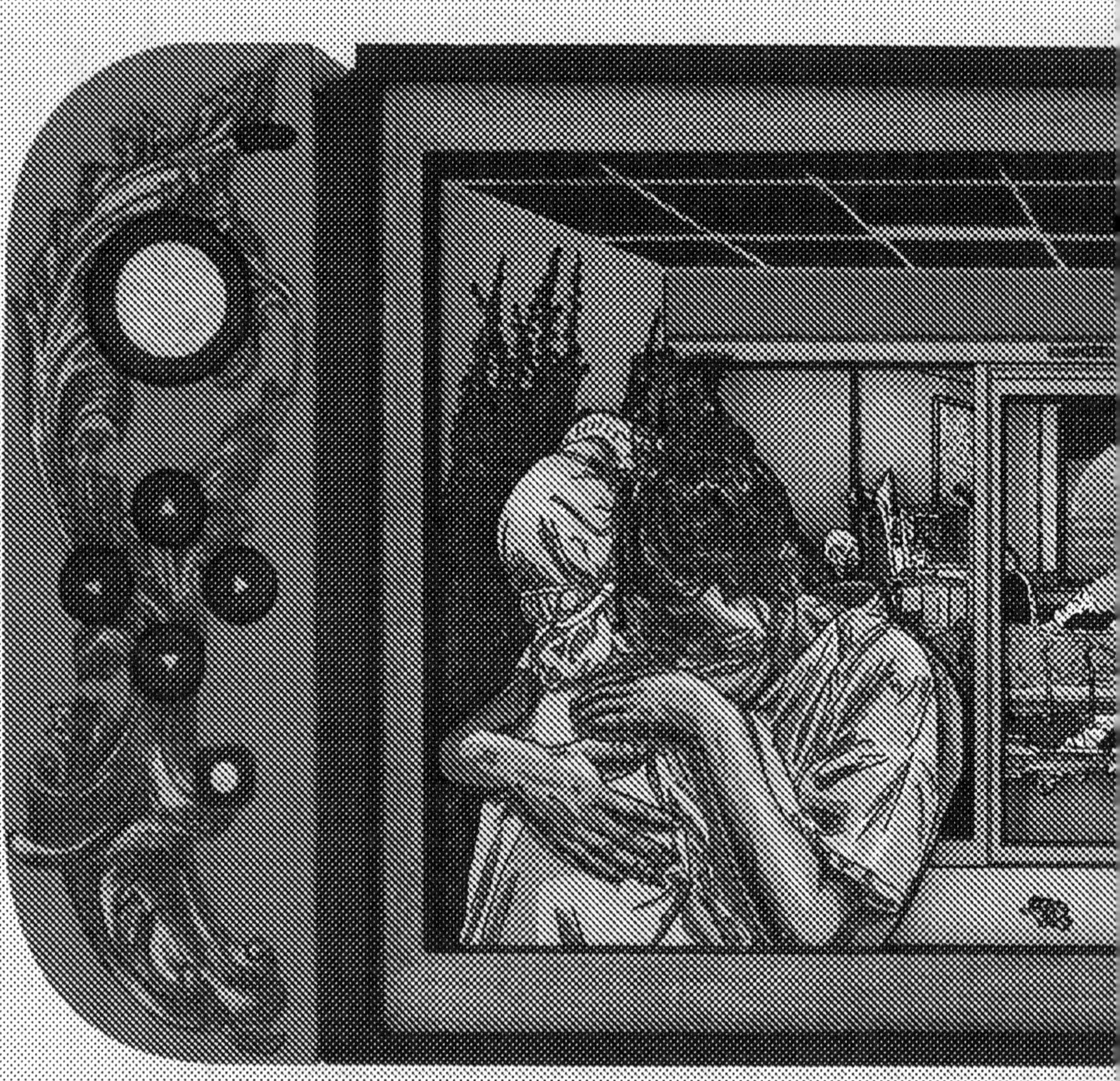

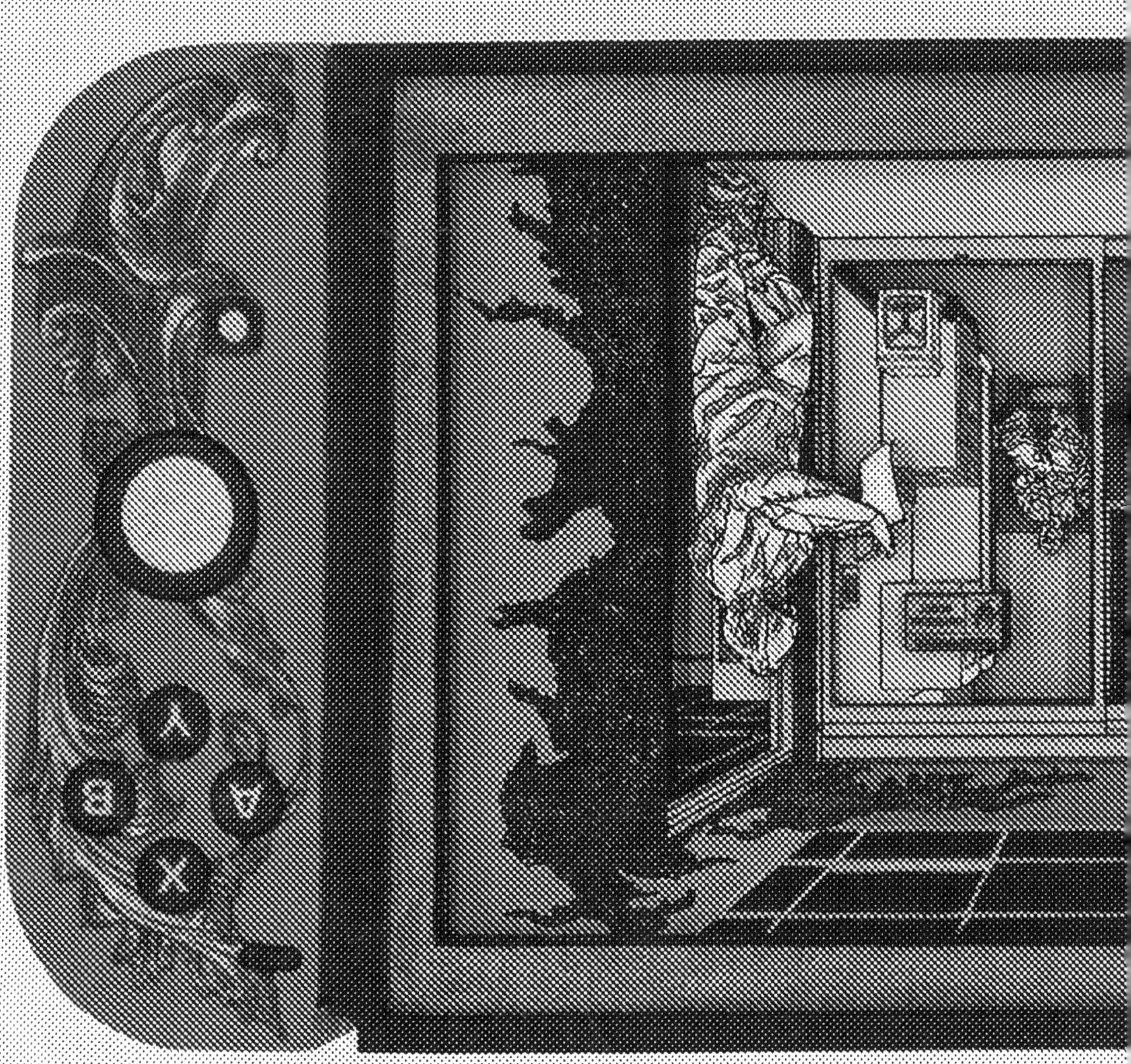

www.ingramcontent.com/pod-product-compliance
Lightning Source LLC
LaVergne TN
LVHW082348100826
845148LV00021B/957